WOMEN'S ISSUES

A CLOSER LOOK AT WOMEN'S HEALTH

WOMEN'S ISSUES

Additional books and e-books in this series can be found on Nova's website under the Series tab.

WOMEN'S ISSUES

A CLOSER LOOK AT WOMEN'S HEALTH

LAKISHA ROBERTS
EDITOR

nova
Medicine & Health
New York

DOI: https://doi.org/10.52305/DBZI4521

NOTICE TO THE READER

Library of Congress Cataloging-in-Publication Data

ISBN: 978-1-68507-408-1

Published by Nova Science Publishers, Inc. † New York

Contents

PREFACE

This book includes six chapters that detail various aspects of women's health. Chapter one uses a hermeneutic phenomenological method to explore hope in eating disordered women. Chapter two considers the importance of hope as a mediating factor in the complicated relationships between body shame and eating disorder behavior as well as with substance use/abuse behavior via an Internet survey. Chapter three examines the influence of six Indigenous Australian sportswomen and their role as sporting role models for women and girls. Chapter four highlights the research that has been conducted regarding eating disorders in women of color and reviews the unique race and culture-related risk factors that may influence the presence of eating disorder symptoms. Chapter five deals with the history and definition of food craving, the cognitive event of appetizing targeting, the associations with the diet mentality as a promoter of moral judgment concerning food, and the twelve primary triggers according to the latest data from studies in the field of eating disorders. Finally, chapter six focuses on the association between physical activity and menopausal transition from the viewpoint of evolutionary biology and evolutionary medicine.

Chapter 1 - This qualitative study used a hermeneutic phenomenological method to explore hope in eating disordered women. Seven women with clinical eating disorders were interviewed in order to understand their experience of hope in a Twelve-Step (12-Step) self-help group. Thematic analysis revealed a three-stage, process-oriented model of the hope in their recovery: (1) Stage 1: Searching for Hope, Removing the Stigma, (2) Stage 2: Sustaining Hope, Receiving Support, and (3) Stage 3: Sharing Hope, Retelling the Story. Three core-themes were embedded within each stage: accepting and understanding, connecting, and trusting. These findings provide a picture of women's experience of hope, suggesting that 12-Step self-help groups can help in their finding, maintaining, and promoting hope, and enhancing their recovery. Implications for practice, notably the importance of hope and hope-focused interventions in eating disorder treatment, are discussed.

Chapter 2 - The eating disorder literature has not adequately considered the importance of hope as a mediating factor in the complicated relationships between body shame and eating disorder behavior, nor its relationship with substance use/abuse behavior. To provide more clarity, an Internet survey of women (N = 297) examined substance use/abuse (alcohol and drugs) as a function of body shame, hope, and eating disorder symptomatology. Twenty-percent reported treatment for an eating disorder at some time; 10% had been treated for anorexia nervosa (AN), with 8.1% treated for bulimia nervosa (BN). Forty-six percent had been treated for both AN and BN. Most had been treated within the last two years (49%), but fully 22% had been treated 6 years or more in the past. Seventy-seven percent of the sample reported alcohol use/abuse, and 76% non-medical drug use/abuse. Structural equation modeling (Lavaan, SEM) tested a series of models, finding that hope and body shame were critical mediators, linking eating disorder symptomatology (EAT-26) to women's alcohol and drug use/abuse behavior. Hope was the dominant factor. Women treated for AN were more impacted by variations in hope. BNs had either direct links to substance use/abuse, or had an effect mediated by eating disorder symptomatology. The implications of these findings for research and practice are discussed.

Chapter 3 - Sporting role models (SRM) can inspire and influence attitude and behavior. This chapter examines the influence of six

Indigenous Australian sportswomen: cricketers Faith Thomas and Ashleigh Gardner, netballers Marcia Ella-Duncan and Jemma MiMi, and tennis players Evonne Goolagong-Cawley and Ashleigh Barty. By applying and extending Marianne Meier's (2015) theoretical lens, it unearths and examines their role as SRMs for women and girls. Meier (2015) recognizes and describes nine functions of SRMs: participation, leadership, advocacy, challenging gender stereotypes, inspiration, ethics, safeguarding and prevention, media and corporates, and giving back. Correspondingly, Meier also identifies three categories on a 'continuum of interaction' between an observer and a successful SRM. Metaphorically the women start in silence; however, the evidence suggests that they gain—and sometimes regain—voice, often beyond their sport careers. Understanding Indigenous sportswomen's SRM status enables a layered and deep understanding of the unique platform provided by sport, which serves to strengthen their influence. The research recognizes a tenth function of female Indigenous SRMs—that of *cultural maintenance*. Findings illuminate how Indigenous Australian sportswomen are constructed in complex and sometimes contradictory ways, at times portrayed as advocates, deviants, sporting ambassadors, and political activists. Further research is needed to untangle the complexities and fluidity of female Indigenous Australian SRMs in the evolving worlds of both professional and community sport.

Chapter 4 - Lack of research examining Women of Color and eating disorders (EDs) can be attributed to the fact that eating disorders were historically considered to occur only in White women. Yet, current research reports have demonstrated that eating disorder symptoms are a significant problem experienced by *all* women, regardless of race and/or ethnicity. The reported incidences of eating disorder symptoms in Women of Color underscore the need for practitioners to know how to effectively assess and treat *all* individuals who struggle with eating, weight, and body image concerns. Since Women of Color may be less likely to receive referrals or to seek treatment for eating disorder symptoms based partially on prevailing stereotypes of traditional eating disorder clients, cultural mistrust of healthcare systems, fear of stigmatization and/or lack of access to resources, practitioners have an ethical responsibility to provide culturally responsive assessment, prevention and treatment for Women of Color. This chapter will highlight briefly the research that has been conducted among Black/African American, Latinx and Asian American women, review the unique race and culture-related risk factors that may influence the presence of eating disorder symptoms in these populations and provide implications for practitioners.

Chapter 5 - One of the aspects involved in the motivation for food consumption and the physiological need for food is Desires for food and Food Cravings. Although there are several definitions for Food Craving in the literature, it is currently understood as a cognitive event involving emotional, physiological, and external aspects. Desires, when intense, also involve torture and awareness of a lack (i.e., Food Craving) which is associated with the diet mentality and cognitive restraint and also associations between affectivity, environment present in Disordered Eating and Eating Disorders cases, which suffer from the greater intensity of Food Craving compared to individuals without Eating Disorders. In this chapter, I deal with the history and definition of Food Craving, the description of the cognitive event of appetizing targeting, the associations with the diet mentality as a promoter of moral judgment concerning food, and the twelve primary triggers (external: positive/negative events, food environment, advertising, cultural beliefs about food, specific places, the food itself and internal triggers: dietary restraint, food reward, impulsivity/inflexibility, emotions/thoughts/feelings about food, hunger/satiety/appetite and finally, anxiety and depression symptoms) according to the latest data from studies in the field of Eating Disorders. Finally, it is the nutritional treatment of Food Cravings in cases of Disordered Eating and Eating Disorders that involve cognitive approaches aimed at eating behavior and the involvement of the principles of Intuitive Eating and the satisfaction of food desires and FC's treatment.

Chapter 6 - Physical activity during menopausal transition is a recommended strategy to reduce climacteric complaints, to prevent obesity, metabolic and cardiovascular diseases but also to avoid accelerated bone loss resulting in long term health hazards such as osteoporosis. The positive effects of physical activity for the prevention of obesity, metabolic and cardiovascular diseases as well as an accelerated reduction of bone density are widely accepted. The effects of physical activity on climacteric symptomatology however, are controversially discussed. From an evolutionary viewpoint, we are designed to be physically active. Therefore, physical activity is not only a treatment strategy, it should be an essential part of our life. The present review focuses on the association between physical activity and menopausal transition from the viewpoint of evolutionary biology and evolutionary medicine.

In: A Closer Look at Women's Health
Editor: Lakisha Roberts
ISBN: 978-1-68507-408-1

Chapter 1

WOMEN'S EXPERIENCE OF HOPE IN A TWELVE-STEP SELF-HELP GROUP FOR EATING DISORDERS

Jennifer A. Boisvert*, PhD
Independent Practice, Beverly Hills, CA, USA

ABSTRACT

This qualitative study used a hermeneutic phenomenological method to explore hope in eating disordered women. Seven women with clinical eating disorders were interviewed in order to understand their experience of hope in a Twelve-Step (12-Step) self-help group. Thematic analysis revealed a three-stage, process-oriented model of the hope in their recovery: (1) Stage 1: Searching for Hope, Removing the Stigma, (2) Stage 2: Sustaining Hope, Receiving Support, and (3) Stage 3: Sharing Hope, Retelling the Story. Three core-themes were embedded within each stage: accepting and understanding, connecting, and trusting. These findings provide a picture of women's experience of hope, suggesting that 12-Step self-help groups can help in their finding, maintaining, and promoting hope, and enhancing their recovery.

* Corresponding Author's E-mail: jenniferboisvert@hotmail.com.

Implications for practice, notably the importance of hope and hope-focused interventions in eating disorder treatment, are discussed.

Keywords: women, eating disorders, hope, recovery, 12-Step groups, self-help groups, treatment

Introduction

The *Diagnostic and Statistical Manual of Mental Disorders* (*DSM-5*: APA, 2013) defines clinical eating disorders as mental disorders that are characterized by extreme disturbances of eating behavior. Anorexia nervosa (AN) is characterized by an extreme fear of weight gain and restrictive eating, while bulimia nervosa (BN) is characterized by bingeing then compensating for having binge eaten through purging, excessive exercise, or fasting behaviors (APA, 2013). AN and BN subtypes reflect an overlapping of symptoms in these eating disorders (APA, 2013).

Eating disorders are multi-dimensional, complex, and chronic illnesses, with biological, sociocultural, and psychological factors all contributing to their development in women (for reviews, see Hesse-Biber et al., 2006; Striegel-Moore & Bulik, 2007). Despite the complexity of eating disorders, they have been widely recognized as "primarily a female psychopathology" (Murnen & Smolak, 2015; Smolak & Murnen, 2001; Striegel-Moore & Bulik, 2007, p. 184). Studies consistently show women are significantly more affected (Lewinsohn et al., 2002; Striegel-Moore et al., 2009). Eating disorders disproportionately affect women, with lifetime prevalence as high as 3:1 compared to men (Fairburn & Harrison, 2003; Hoek, 2006; Hoek & van Hoeken, 2003; Hudson et al., 2007). However, research has also documented eating disorder symptomatology in men (Boisvert & Harrell, 2009a, 2009b, 2012). Eating disorders are the third most common chronic illness among adolescents and young adult women in the United States, having reached the point of a "social epidemic" in these populations (Gordon, 2000).

Eating disorders are regarded as unremitting, with high rates of chronicity and mortality, and have been linked to serious medical complications and psychosocial disturbances (Klein & Walsh, 2004; Rome & Ammerman, 2003; Williamson et al., 2004). In both AN and BN women, risk for mortality increases with longer duration of illness, lower body mass index (BMI), alcohol and drug use, and poorer psychosocial functioning (Franko et al., 2013). In AN women, there are higher rates of mortality (Arcelus et al., 2011; Herzog et al., 2000; Hoek, 2006). These women tend to be highly treatment resistant, and, thus, fail to engage in treatment or drop-out prematurely (Abbate-Daga et al., 2015; for review, see Abbate-Daga et al., 2013). Practitioners might view patients who "fail to change" as "treatment-resistant cases" with little to no hope for improvement or recovery (for review, see Wonderlich et al., 2012, p. 467). These women often die from medical complications or suicide as they tend to have a higher desire to die and use more severe, lethal methods than BN women or non-eating disordered women (Arcelus et al., 2011; Forcano et al., 2011; Guillaume et al., 2011).

Lack of hope, i.e., hopelessness, has been linked to depression, social disconnection, and suicidal ideation and attempts (Herrestad, & Biong, 2010; Huen et al., 2015). Increasing hope, i.e., hopefulness, might be a promising intervention for reducing self-harm behavior, particularly suicidality, but possibly, too, eating disorder symptomatology.

Hope and Eating Disorder Symptomatology

Hope is the belief that one's goals can be met in the future (Herth, 1991). A higher level of hope, i.e., hopefulness, can help a person in meeting a future goal(s) and experiencing health benefits such as wholeness (Herth, 1991). Hope is believed to play a critical role in enhancing optimal health and well-being, and promoting adaptive processes, including recovering from or rising above the adversity of chronic illness (Nekolaichuk, 1995; Nekolaichuck & Bruera, 1998; Nekolaichuk et al., 1999). Hope is a multi-dimensional, experiential process involving future- and action-orientation, realism, positive expectation, uncertainty, intentionality or agency, and interconnection with self/others (Doe, 2019; Morse & Doberneck, 1995; Morse & Penrod, 1999).

In Herth's (1987, 1989, 1991, 1992) model, hope is conceptualized as a dynamic process comprising three dimensions: (a) action-oriented and process-oriented, (b) thoughts, feelings, and behaviors that change over time and circumstances, and (c) interconnectedness derived from spiritual and social resources. Herth theorized that a person's level of hope is reflective of her strengths or deficits in three domains. These three domains are: (1) cognitive-temporal – a perception that a positive desired outcome is realistically probable in the near or distant future, (2) affective-behavioral – a feeling of confidence with initiation of plans to affect the desired outcome expressed as a sense of positive readiness and expectancy, and (3) affiliative-contextual – a recognition of an interconnectedness between self and others, including a higher spiritual power (e.g., God). In Herth's model, hope as a process is experienced by persons on a global or specific level, being influenced by individual and/or situational factors (Farran et al., 1995).

Studies support Herth's model of hope as multi-dimensional, with level of hope varying due to individual factors (e.g., health status) and/or situational factors (e.g., environment) (Buckley & Herth, 2004; Herth, 1990, 1993, 1996; Vandecreek et al., 1994). Level of hope has been identified as a key factor in psychological and physical health, with lower hope associated with greater psychological and physical problems (Buckley & Herth, 2004; Herth, 1987, 1989, 1991, 1990, 1993, 1996; Vandecreek et al., 1994). More recently, the investigation of Herth's model, i.e., level of hope, relative to health has extended to eating disorder symptomatology.

Boisvert (2001, 2006) and Boisvert and Harrell (2013a, 2016a), as part of their research program on eating disorders, conducted several studies exploring relationships between level of hope and eating disorder symptomatology in clinical and nonclinical women. Using Herth's (1991) model of hope and corresponding scales/indices (HHS/HHI: Herth, 1991, 1992) in these studies, the results identified lower hope as a risk factor for eating disorder symptomatology.

Boisvert (2001) investigated the relationship between level of hope and symptom severity in eating disordered women. A clinical sample eating disordered women (N = 31; AN n = 17, BN n = 14) and a comparison sample of nonclinical women (N = 31) completed a questionnaire of standardized, self-report measures on hope and eating disorder symptomatology. Hope was measured using the Herth Hope Scale (HHS: Herth, 1991). T-tests showed that compared to nonclinical women, eating disordered women had lower hope in general, and specifically, lower interconnectedness, and lower positive readiness and expectancy. Correlation analyses showed a relationship of lower hope and greater eating disorder symptom severity in general, and specific to symptoms of social insecurity, ineffectiveness, and interpersonal distrust.

Boisvert (2006) examined relationships between hope and eating disorder symptomatology in a sample of nonclinical women (N = 641). Correlation analyses revealed lower hope was associated with greater body shame and eating disorder symptomatology. Path analyses showed a direct effect of hope on eating disorder symptomatology and indirect effects of hope on eating disorder symptomatology. Body shame mediated the indirect effects of hope on eating disorder symptomatology. Hope was also found to mediate the relationships between spirituality and eating disorder symptomatology.

Boisvert and Harrell (2013a) investigated the effects of hope, body shame, and body mass index (BMI) on eating disorder symptomatology in a sample of nonclinical women (N = 641). ANOVA analyses revealed strong main effects of BMI, body shame, and hope. In general, body shame was more likely to be reported by women above the medians on BMI and body shame and below the median on hope. Hopefulness was a significant moderating variable, lowering eating disorder symptomatology for women with high BMI and body shame.

Boisvert and Harrell (2016a) examined relationships between hope, perfectionism, ineffectiveness, spirituality, body dissatisfaction, and eating disorder symptomatology in a nonclinical sample of women (N = 642). Path analyses showed hope had a strong indirect effect on eating disorder symptomatology, specifically drive for thinness and bulimia. Higher hope women perceived themselves to be less ineffective, with lower body dissatisfaction and lower drive for thinness and bulimia.

Altogether, this suggests that lower hope can make women vulnerable to developing eating disorder symptomatology, having greater symptomatology severity, or be a barrier to their successful treatment and recovery. In this chapter, we will find that the experience of hope by eating disordered women sheds light on its importance for recovery.

Hope and Recovery

Eating disorder recovery has been described by women as a cyclic process of accepting the disease, accepting self and others, accepting spirituality, having a sense of self-worth, thinking more rationally, relinquishing struggle for control (over food/body weight), and re-joining society (D'Abdundo & Chally, 2004; for reviews, see de Vos et al., 2017; Espíndola & Blay, 2009). Qualitative studies of AN and BN women in recovery have identified themes of accepting oneself and the body, awareness and tolerance of negative emotions, developing and maintaining supportive relationships, self-empowerment, self-determined search for identity and truth, and becoming "whole" again (Björk & Ahlström, 2008; Federici & Kaplan, 2008; Jenkins & Ogden, 2012; Nordbø et al., 2008; for reviews, see Duncan et al., 2015; Wetzler et al., 2020).

Emphasizing the cyclic process of recovery are studies featuring descriptions of its nonlinear nature, and depictions of it as a visual model with circular stages/phases. A study of eating disordered adolescent girls (N = 10) content analyzed interviews to uncover metaphors of change, with recovery described as a "journey" of getting to know themselves better, with this journey "going forward and backward and up and down" (Mathieson & Hoskins, 2005, p. 268).

Björk and Ahlström (2008) conducted a study of the experience of recovery in AN and BN women (and eating disorder not otherwise specified [EDNOS]) (*N* = 14) using open-ended interviews. Thematic analysis revealed recovery was experienced in various ways, with four categories describing being more relaxed and accepting of food/eating behavior, the body, themselves as persons (including permitting and dealing with emotions), and attending to social relations.

Similarly, in a study of BN women's (*N* = 14) experience of recovery, Lindgren et al., (2015) used open-ended interviews and content analysis, showing recovery, via a visual model, as a four-stage process with subthemes of: hitting bottom and opening up about the illness, searching for a new identity, accepting help and doing the work, feeling valuable as a person, and feeling free of BN.

With respect to hope in recovery, there is recognition that "…the central tenet in recovery is hope—it is the catalyst for change, and the enabler of the other factors involved in recovery to take charge" (Acharya & Agius, 2017, p. S619). When hope (or hopelessness) is mentioned, it is brief and in reference to other factors facilitating recovery (Arthur-Cameselle & Baltzell, 2012; Dawson et al., 2014; Hannon et al., 2017; Hay & Cho, 2013; Higginson & Mansell, 2008; Ibrahim & Tchanturia, 2018; Las Hayas et al., 2016; Wright & Hacking, 2012; for review, see Wetzler et al., 2020). For example, Hannon et al. (2017) explored the experience of illness, treatment, and change in AN women (*N* = 8), identifying a theme of "hopelessness versus hope," but described it in relation to longer treatment with little or no change, thus, hopelessly "stuck."

There has been no in-depth exploration of hope in eating disordered women except for a study by Boisvert (2003). In this study, Boisvert (2003) chronicled an anorexic women's experience of hope in recovery using heuristic case study and visual/textual media, e.g., photography, journal entries, poems (see also Boisvert, 2012a). Content and thematic analyses identified four metaphors and themes: (1) opening the shutter (liberty)—photography gave a reason to hope for a more liberating existence, (2) focusing the lens (security)—photography as a form of risk-taking, enabling a sense of security in navigating the inner world, (3) framing the image (reality)—photography as re-framing self-perceptions and seeing reality, and (4) taking the picture (vitality)—photography as capturing a picture of hope for the future and offering self-healing. These themes reflect a paralleling of hope and recovery processes, and the use of photography to promote these processes. The creation of a visual diary was found to enhance metaphoric self-understanding and the development of a healthier self, a "hopeful self-healer identity" (Boisvert, 2003, p. 28).

Twelve-Step (12-Step) Self-Help Groups

Qualitative research has identified the importance of supportive relationships with other eating disordered sufferers for recovery (Beveridge et al., 2019; Nicholls et al., 2016; for reviews, see Bell, 2003; Bezance & Holliday, 2013; Wetzler et al., 2020). Specific themes identified were inspiration gained from receiving support from another sufferer, the value of a collaborative, equal, reciprocal power dynamic, and instillation of hope for recovery (Beveridge et al., 2019; Nicholls et al., 2016). Other qualitative data suggest supportive relationships amongst sufferers in self-help groups facilitate recovery (Button & Warren, 2001; de la Rie et al., 2006; Hsu et al., 1992; Noordenbos, 1989; Rorty et al., 1993; for review, see Bell, 2003).

For example, Pivarunas (2016) explored the experience of a religious faith-based support group for women with disordered eating (N = 5). Participants' written responses to open-ended questions identified a need for relational growth in their relationship with God and others, and that they experienced connectedness and hope.

Twelve-Step (12-Step) self-help groups are typically used as an adjunct in the treatment of eating disorders and other addictions such as alcohol and/or drug use (von Ranson & Farstad, 2014). The text,

Alcoholics Anonymous (AA) (the "Big Book": AA World Services, 1939), outlines the AA 12-Step program while its companion text, *Twelve Steps and Twelve Traditions* (AA World Services, 1952) elaborates on the 12-Step philosophy. In 12-Step programs, "These steps are worked not just once as an act of salvation, but rather as an ongoing lifelong program for living. Sobriety is similarly understood in a spiritual context, involving far more than being abstinent...[it is] having to do with a spiritual maturity that involves acceptance, humility and serenity" (Miller, 1998, p. 981). This program is truly one of the few places in contemporary life where people can be "real" in honestly sharing their weaknesses, failings, character defects, imperfections, humanness, and meet a need for self/social identity (Khantzian & Mack, 1994).

As a "spiritual recovery movement," 12-Step programs use group processes that engage its members in behavioral expectations associated with their health issues, and interrupt and modify core problems in self-regulation (Galanter, 2007; Khantzian & Mack, 1994). "Working the Steps" promotes a "spiritual awakening" and changes views of the "addiction," helping recovering persons practice the 12-Steps and principles of the fellowship in their daily affairs, and carry the message to others (Green et al., 1998; Steigerwald & Stone, 1999).

Overeaters Anonymous (OA) is the most widely known application of the 12-Step philosophy to compulsive overeaters, i.e., binge eating, with membership requiring a desire to stop eating compulsively (OA, 1990). OA members often report compulsive overeating and a range of dysfunctional eating patterns, including BN, for which they seek help in OA (Russell-Mayhew et al., 2010; von Ranson et al., 2011; Wasson, 2003; Wasson & Jackson, 2004).

Research on OA offers a glimpse of how it is helpful or effective for its members. Wasson and Jackson (2004) conducted a study exploring the role of OA in member's treatment experiences. Women with BN (N = 26) attending OA for six months or more were engaged in semi-structured interviews along with four focus group sessions. Analysis revealed that participants used five OA skills or strategies. According to Wasson and Jackson (2004): "These included: (1) OA meeting attendance and participation, (2) interaction with a sponsor, (3) processing (i.e., writing and journaling), (4) spirituality (i.e., prayer and meditation), and (5) adherence to a food plan" (p. 337). Specifically, Wasson and Jackson (2004), state: "Regular meeting attendance benefited members by (1) providing instruction for using the Twelve Steps; (2) decreasing feelings of isolation through sharing feelings with others with similar eating concerns; (3) reducing feelings of self-criticism and instilling hope for recovery; and (4) facilitating members to identify and articulate the behavior patterns involved in their binge eating or purging" (p. 351). The majority of participants described "…spirituality as the core of their recovery…[and that] members in this study appreciated that the [OA] program did not define or prescribe a specific belief in a higher power and instead offered members the freedom to develop their personal concept" (p. 352).

Russell-Mayhew et al. (2010) conducted a study exploring member's experiences and perceptions of OA. Women (n = 20) and men (n = 1) attending OA (duration unknown) were involved in three focus group sessions. Analysis revealed that participants found a number of 12-Step "tools" were helpful. Explicit "tools" included "…spirituality, OA wisdom, tailoring, abstinence, the 12-steps, writing, reaching out, daily readings, meetings, anonymity, service and sponsorship" (p. 37). Implicit "tools" included "…modeling, connection to others, sense of community and honest feedback to self and others" (p. 37). According to Russell-Mayhew et al. (2010), "The spiritual nature of the program was experienced as different from any other available program…Participants emphasized that if there was one tool that was most helpful, it was the spiritual nature of OA" (p. 37). Participants reported that OA's framing the compulsive overeating as an addiction offered them a new way of seeing their problem, and this principle and OA's emphasis on the emotional and spiritual aspects of recovery made OA effective.

Hertz, Addad, and Ronel (2012) conducted a study on OA members' recovery. Women with binge eating disorder (N = 20) attending OA for a year were engaged in semi-structured, in-depth interviews. Thematic analysis revealed that the 12-Step "tools" used for spiritual and "emotional work" in OA were essential to recovery. The "secure environment" of OA meetings led to "secure relationships" between group members, reducing their fear of rejection and feelings of loneliness and social exclusion. OA members became securely attached "...when given optimal conditions of love, acceptance, empathy, and the maintenance of equality" (Hertz et al., 2012, p. 118). The spiritual aspect of OA, that is, "...their faith in God's unconditional love of the universe" also helped them recover (Hertz et al., 2012, p. 117).

Ronel and Libman (2003) conducted a study of the experience of compulsive overeating and recovery in OA members. Open-ended interviews were undertaken with women (n = 80) and men (n = 8) who attended OA for some time (few months to several years). Thematic analysis revealed that participants underwent "a world-view transformation" of recovery in four areas: (1) experience of self, (2) universal order/God, (3) relations with others, and (4) perception of the problem. Participants reported their relationships with other OA members were close and sharing. Ronel and Libman (2003) observe: "Sharing the weaknesses, the vulnerability, and the very difficult situations encountered by everyone in the group, creates an atmosphere of understanding, identification, and love, even if unspoken" (p. 164). Recovery was believed to be a constant process of spiritual change, taking personal responsibility for one's "sobriety," and having a social life involving OA members and a relationship to a Higher Power.

Anorexics and Bulimics Anonymous (ABA) applies the 12-Step philosophy to AN and BN, with membership requiring a desire to stop unhealthy eating (ABA, 2002). ABA defines "addiction" as dysfunctional practices that allow members to feel in control of food, weight, and/or body shape (ABA, 2002). ABA members are encouraged to obtain "meal support" from an ABA sponsor (or outside professional, e.g., dietician, nutritionist) planning, preparing, and/or serving all meals and snacks so they are "no longer afraid of getting fat" (ABA, 2002). In ABA, "sobriety" is defined as surrendering to the way that one's Higher Power wants them to eat and nourish the body, and accepting the body that one's Higher Power wants them to have (ABA, 2002).

There is no known study of ABA as a self-help group functioning in the community; there is only a single study of an ABA-focused treatment program. Boisvert and Harrell (2016b) conducted a telephone-interview survey of clinical eating disordered women ($N = 22$) who attended a 12-Step approach treatment program to evaluate patient's perceptions of its effectiveness and spiritual benefits. Demographic and correlation analyses showed strong evidence that this program successfully treated a range of eating disordered women, particularly those with AN. Much of its success was due to the strong social connections developed during treatment—something inherent in the 12-Step model and often lacking in traditional medical treatments. While hope was not specifically examined, the participants indicated that the strong social ties of the 12-Step program were helpful for promoting recovery, suggesting that interconnectedness as a facet of hope might have been experienced.

Purpose of the Study

The purpose of the study reported in this chapter is to explore eating disordered women's experience of hope in a 12-Step self-help group for eating disorders. It aimed at understanding the meaning of hope for women in the context of group participation, and the importance of hope for recovery. It is believed that practitioner's greater understanding of how 12-Step self-help group interaction process can enhance hope and, hence, recovery, will encourage them to use hope-focused interventions.

METHOD

Research Design

A qualitative research approach was used because it has two important characteristics. First, there is emphasis on subjectivity when examining human realities and truths. As such, the researcher is integral to the study, and is, in fact, the research instrument rather than objective observer. Second, there is emphasis on understanding experiences as a whole and within its rich context. As a result, it is less reductive in its data analysis than is a quantitative approach. Overall, this approach is used to document the subjective, experiential life-world of human beings, offering a description of their experiences in-depth (Patton, 2002).

A Hermeneutic Phenomenological Approach

A hermeneutic phenomenological method of inquiry was used to explore eating disordered women's experience of hope in a 12-Step self-help group. This methodology can help practitioners more clearly understand the importance of hope as a process enhancing recovery from eating disorders from the participant's point of view. This clarity is missing in the professional helping literature. Having a clear awareness of how these women experience hope can inform a practitioner's use of interventions for increasing hope and decreasing eating disorder and other self-destructive behavior, including suicidality, which has been linked to hopelessness.

As a descriptive methodology, phenomenology aspires to describe and clarify the essential structures of human phenomena, that is, lived experience or the life-world (van Manen, 1997). Hermeneutics, through interpretation and insight, intend to uncover the meaning of human phenomena, elucidating the lived world in a way that expands our understanding of human experience and human being (van Manen, 1997). Hermeneutic phenomenology focuses on the interpretation of the life-world or human experience as it is lived, and with how things are understood by people who live through these experiences and by those who study them (van Manen, 1977, 1997). Hermeneutic phenomenology, as an interpretive methodology, uses in-depth, layered reflection by the researcher and rich, descriptive language in interview transcripts to reveal the meaning of human experience in a more holistic manner (van Manen, 1997).

Sample

Participants were recruited from a Twelve-Step (12-Step) self-help group in Edmonton, Alberta, Canada. The 12-Step self-help group was based on an addiction model of recovery—Anorexics and Bulimics Anonymous (ABA) (ABA, 2002). This ABA 12-Step approach was adopted based on the founders' personal beliefs and experiences of the 12-Step addiction model as being effective. (As noted above, an ABA 12-Step approach treatment program set up by the founding group members effectively treated clinical eating disorders in women; see Boisvert & Harrell, 2016b.)

The group was comprised of ~15-20 adult women with self-reported clinical eating disorders in various stages of illness and recovery, from acutely ill to full recovery. Group meetings were attended by ~7-10 eating disordered women, informally facilitated by a member, and held weekly (1.5-2 hours) in a community or private setting, e.g., house or church basement. Group members were encouraged to access support through outreach phone calls, sponsor-sponsee meetings, or 12-Step meetings in the community (especially those with addictions of alcohol and/or drug use).

Study participants were seven women who self-reported a clinical eating disorder. Participants had been treated by a medical and/or mental health practitioner, and diagnosed with a clinical eating disorder of AN or BN, or a combination thereof (or a subtype of either). Two women had AN, two women had BN, and three women had a combination of AN and BN. Participant's duration of illness ranged from 9 to 30 years (average 19 years). Participant's duration of recovery ranged from <1 to 14 years (average 5 years).

Participants reported treatment histories of repeated hospitalizations for medical stabilization (n = 6), a specialized eating disorder treatment center (n = 1), and psychotherapy (n = 7). Participants reported being hospitalized 1 to 6 times (average 3 times). Participants reported being in psychotherapy 6 months to 16 years (average 4 years).

Participation in the 12-Step self-help group thus offered an alternative approach to earlier traditional treatment approaches. Participant's group attendance ranged from 6 months to 5 years (average 2 years). Some women had attended other 12-Step self-help groups before, including Overeaters Anonymous (n = 1), Alcoholics Anonymous (AA) (n = 1), and Narcotics Anonymous (NA) (n = 1). Women reported addiction histories of alcohol (n = 2), drugs (n = 1), and alcohol and drugs (n = 2). Participants reported attending the ABA 12-Step group and other 12-Step group meetings from 1 to 4 times per week (average 2 times per week).

Participants ranged in age from 22 to 53 years (average age 37 years). The majority of participants were White (n = 6), with the exception of a single woman of color (East Indian). Women were nearly equally split in marital status: single (n = 3), married (n = 2), and divorced (n = 2). Nearly all women had a post-secondary education (n = 6) and were employed (n = 5), except a woman who was on medical disability because of her eating disorder. The majority of participants reported involvement in eating disorders awareness/activism (n = 5).

The in-depth nature of qualitative inquiry necessitates the use of a small sample. This limits the generalizability of findings, but more fully captures human phenomena that are not easily quantified (Patton, 2002). Participants were recruited through purposeful and snowball sampling. According to Patton (2002), the logic of purposeful sampling lies in its ability to assist the researcher in locating information-rich key informants for detailed study. The following criteria were used to select informants for the study: (a) a self-reported clinical eating disorder of AN or BN (or a subtype), (b) regular attendance, participating in the 12-Step self-help group for a period of at least six months, (c) 18 years of age or older, (d) English-speaking, and (e) female.

Data Collection

Methods of data collection included observation and semi-structured, in-depth interviews. These methods were chosen because they are aligned with hermeneutic phenomenology methodology, granting the researcher first-hand access to participant's lived experiences in different ways.

Observation

The 12-Step self-help group was "underground," accessed by group member invitation. To gain entry, the researcher disclosed her personal and research interests to a group member. Thereafter, the researcher spent considerable time in fieldwork; regularly attending group meetings before, during, and after the study was conducted. This fieldwork provided her contextual information about the 12-Step self-help group (format, processes, and dynamics), and aided her selection of participants based on inclusion criteria. The researcher's group attendance was in accord with Reinharz's (1992) recommendation that the researcher be a member of the group being studied. Observation was used to prompt participants to explore or reflect upon their experiences in interviews, and provide points of reference for interpretation of findings.

Interviews

The interview serves very specific purposes. First, it is used as a means for exploring and gathering narratives or stories of experience. Second, it is a vehicle to develop a conversational relationship with the participant about the meaning of an experience. This may be achieved through reflection with the participant on the topic at hand (van Manen, 1997).

As a reflexive qualitative method, hermeneutic phenomenology prizes the interactive nature of data collection, with findings emerging from the interactions between the researcher and participants as the research progresses (van Manen, 1997). The researcher enters into a "complementary relationship" with participants, establishing trust and rapport to encourage authentic dialogue best capturing their experience, e.g., use of metaphors (Denzin & Lincoln, 1998). As a group member, the researcher disclosed her personal experience (see Boisvert, 2003, 2012a). Participant's awareness of this crucial piece of information about the researcher, and ability to see her as a group "insider" with a shared experience, was expected to foster genuine openness in interviews, and, in turn, enhance robustness of findings (Reinharz, 1992).

Ethical approval was received from the Institutional Review Board (IRB) at the University of Alberta. Verbal and written informed consent was obtained from all participants. Maintaining participant's confidentiality is a major ethical concern of the interpretive research paradigm because of the personal nature of the research and intimate questions. Confidentiality was maintained through the use of participant numbers and pseudonyms (self-chosen by the participants), and by omitting specific contextual details that might reveal participant's identities (Denzin & Lincoln, 1998).

After securing ethical requirements, a single, in-depth, semi-structured interview was conducted with each participant (1-2 hours). Semi-structured interviews provide greater breadth or richness in data than do structured interviews, and allow participants freedom to respond to questions and probes, and to narrate their experiences without being tied down to specific answers (Morse & Field, 1995). A further advantage over unstructured interviews is the ability to compare across interviews due to the consistency of questions asked (Morse & Field, 1995).

Six interviews were conducted in the women's homes and one was conducted in a private office. Questions were designed to explore participant's experience within three areas of concentration: (a) the experience of having an eating disorder, (b) the experience of participating in the 12-Step self-help group, and (c) the experience of hope. All interviews were audio-recorded and transcribed verbatim by the researcher so there was full immersion in the data (van Manen, 1997).

To ensure saturation of the data, interviews were conducted until thematic repetition in the transcripts was noted and participants reported they had no new information to offer. No new categories emerged by the fifth interview. However, two more interviews were conducted to ensure that the data were rich and varied, in addition to being saturated.

Data Analysis

Data analysis involved thematic analysis using a hermeneutic phenomenological method described by van Manen (1997). Phenomenological themes may be understood as "structures of experience" (or "meaning units"), which are identified by reading and re-reading all transcripts then taking a holistic theme from each individual transcript (van Manen, 1997). This process of familiarizing oneself with the data (via listening and reading) is often referred to as "immersion" (in the data) (van Manen, 1997). It involves engaging with the meaning of the transcripts in order to get a "sense" or preliminary interpretation of them (van Manen, 1997). This is followed by a selective "highlighting" approach to statements or phrases throughout the transcript (van Manen, 1997). The themes or subthemes that are identified in the text become objects for further reflection and interpretation (van Manen, 1997). van Manen (1997) suggests that when description is mediation by expression, including nonverbal aspects, e.g., silences, a stronger element of interpretation is involved. These isolated phenomenal themes are then re-written with an attendant interpretation that was written above or below the extracted statement, while also interpreting the meaning of the phenomenon or lived experience (van Manen, 1997). van Manen's (1997) "existentials," which are theme types that act as guides for reflection in analysis, were used: (a) lived space—"spaciality," (b) lived body—corporality, (c) lived time—temporality, and lived human relation—

"relationality." These themes may be seen as a reflection of the existential way that humans experience the life-world (van Manen, 1997).

Participant's actual words in the form of quotations are used to demonstrate the structures of experience (i.e., the raw data, unadulterated by the researcher's interpretation of it), and offer examples based on interpretation. The selection of participant's thematic statements was guided by what constitutes quality data per van Manen (1997). In reporting the findings, van Manen (1990) states: "Phenomenology, not unlike poetry, is a poetizing project: it tries an incantative, evocative speaking, a primal telling, wherein we aim to involve the voice in an original singing of the world" (p. 13). van Manen (2007) states this reporting should be a balance of science-art.

Ensuring Quality of Data

To ensure quality, the researcher selected criteria that were consistent with the research design (Lincoln & Guba, 2000; Patton, 2002). Several strategies have been identified in the literature as enhancing trustworthiness of the findings (or "rigor" as termed by Guba & Lincoln, 1981), including congruence between the research design and methods used, prolonged engagement with the participants and the phenomena, multiple methods of data collected, and auditable records (Guba & Lincoln, 1982; Lincoln & Guba, 2000; Patton, 2002).

Data were collected over a period of several months, allowing opportunity to observe the group beforehand, establish rapport with participants, gain trust, and be regarded as an "insider." Multiple methods and sources of data collection provide multiple constructions of phenomena, enhancing the depth and richness of the data and reducing systematic bias (Lincoln & Guba, 2000). Further, it encourages reflexivity in data collection and analysis, sensitivity to the research data in analysis, and transparency of the research process (Reinharz, 1992). Methods used included documenting written interview transcripts, memoing, writing field notes, creating an audit trail, and developing a mind map of the themes. Various sources on eating disorders, group processes, and hope (e.g., scholarly books, articles, conferences, videos) enabled data interpretation to be cross-referenced and validated (Guba, 1981; Lincoln & Guba, 2000).

Credibility refers to the vividness and faithfulness of the description of the phenomenon (Guba & Lincoln, 1982), or trustworthiness of the findings (Denzin & Lincoln, 2000). Authenticity is demonstrated if researchers show a range of different realities in a fair and balanced manner (fairness) (Denzin & Lincoln, 1998). Using multiple methods and sources of data collection strengthens the claim that the researcher dealt fairly with these. To be fair, a quotation from each participant is presented in the Results so that each unique "voice" is heard.

Ensuring that participant's voices (and that of the researcher) are present in the text also enhanced authenticity (Lincoln & Guba, 2000). This was achieved by using rich descriptions and participant's words to allow them to speak for themselves (Guba & Lincoln, 1982). Each participant's "voice" was used to reflect different viewpoints.

The veracity of the findings was established through member checking (Guba & Lincoln, 1982). Credibility of the findings was enhanced by seeking two participant's reactions to, elaboration of, and corroboration of emergent categories and themes in a 1:1 meeting (≥ 1 hour). The confirmability and transferability of the findings were established through external checks (Guba, 1981; Guba & Lincoln, 1982). External readers who offered feedback on the findings included a non-participant group member in a 1:1 meeting (≥ 1 hour) and multiple meetings/exchanges with colleagues with expertise in the topic of study.

RESULTS

Hope was integral to the recovery process for women in the 12-Step self-help group. Thematic analysis of participant's descriptions of group interactions revealed a three-stage, process-oriented model of hope: (1) Stage 1: Searching for Hope and Removing the Stigma, (2) Stage 2:

Sustaining Hope and Receiving Support, and (3) Stage 3: Sharing Hope and Retelling the Story (see Figure 1). Three core-themes were embedded within each stage: accepting and understanding, connecting, and trusting (see Figure 2). The core-themes capture common aspects across and within participant's experiences, reflecting the experience of hope as a dynamic *process*. Participant interviews revealed that stages of the model could be accessed and re-accessed cyclically.

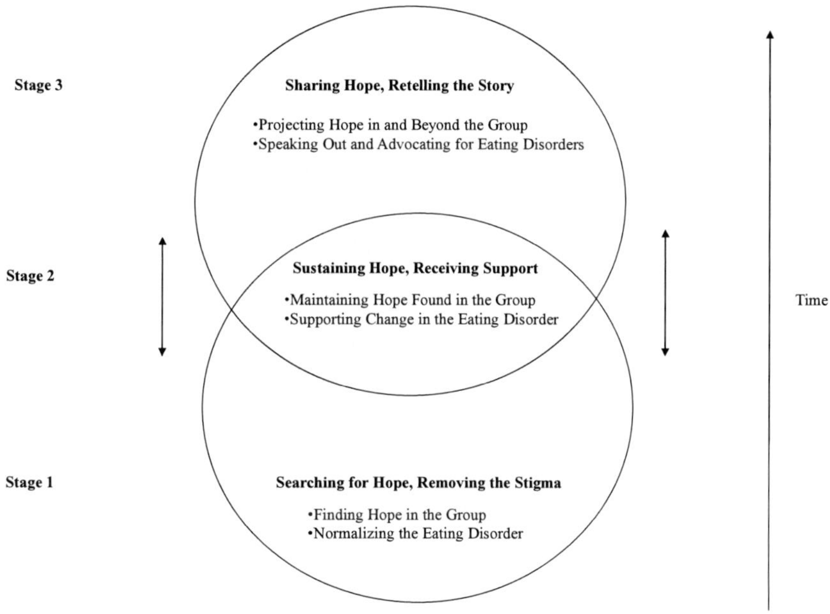

Figure 1. A model of hope as a process.

Figure 1 depicts this re-accessing of hope by the overlapping of stages. Similarly, the model uses terms (i.e., hop*ing*) to convey semantically that the experience of hope is a process involving movement between the stages, indicative of growth (Farran et al., 1995). Figure 1 depicts this hoping process as moving women forward, furthering their recovery over time by an upward arrow.

Certainly, there are no words more powerful than those of the women themselves to describe the meaning of the experience of hope. Below, in each of the three stages, participant quotes illustrate each of the three core-themes.

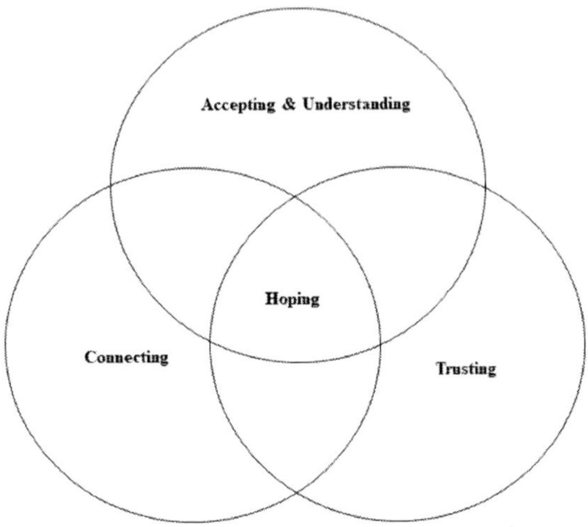

Figure 2. Core-themes of the experience of hope as a process.

Stage 1: Searching for Hope, Removing the Stigma

The first stage reflects participant's experience of *searching for hope* before attending the group. Hope was found when others normalized their eating disorder. It was experienced through bearing witness to others' lived experiences, and developing trust in the group space. *Removing the stigma* and shame of their disorder was particularly important to discovering hope.

In this stage (and next two stages), hope was an opening pointing towards a future vision. The women regarded hope as a sense of inner peace, tranquility, and serenity, describing it as disentangling themselves from the eating disorder. It was clear that hope meant freeing oneself from the "insanity" or "obsession" of eating disordered behaviors. This reflected the 12-Step program aim of lessening addiction and maintaining "sobriety." There was expectancy that despite their past or present self-destructive eating disordered behaviors, they were going to be "OK" in coming out of their near-death experiences alive. There was an overall sense of "we can live with hope" and "hope is a sign of recovery."

> "Hope…is…that feeling that things are going to be OK. Hope that…that I'll…that I-I'm not, I guess gonna [die]. That I'll, I'll keep on living, and, and that uh, …gives me a sense of serenity I guess. And peacefulness, and that life's OK…I have that sense of, you know, peacefulness or serenity…that's my hope. And uh, that things will continue on positively." [Participant 1, "Michelle"]

Stage 1 core-themes of the hoping process are outlined below.

"People Accept Me for Who I Am"

Hope arose from participant's feeling accepted and understood by the group. Other's normalizing their eating disorder experience helped them to accept and understand their eating disorder *as a disorder* that was separate from them *as a person*. There was hope being in the company of others who knew first-hand what it meant to diet, starve, purge, or engage in other "addictive," self-destructive eating disordered behaviors. The feeling of being non-pathologized and known as persons could *only* come from the group—from one "addict" to another "addict." This was a cornerstone of the 12-Step program. Participants spoke of how they were in "hiding" before the group. Family members, friends, or clinicians, could not relate to their problem. This lack of understanding led them to feel abnormal and stigmatized, like "freaks," misfits, and lunatics. It also led to feeling disconnected, isolated, depressed, despair, hopelessness, and a wish to die or be dead. Rather than being cured, despair or hopelessness arose from a series of unhelpful, "harmful," or failed medical treatments such as hospitalization or behavioral therapy emphasizing weight gain that these women were subject to involuntarily or voluntarily.

> "Um…but, I always come away [from group meetings] with a feeling that I'm going to be OK. That there's people that care about me unconditionally. And it doesn't matter if I come home and put my supper in the toilet. There's still going to be people there that care about me. Whether I've done something like that or not. That they are going to accept me for who I am. And I think that's, I mean, I can't even say that that's important. It's like a lifeline. It's more than just important, it's a lifeline." [Participant 4, "Marie"]

"People Were Telling My Story"

Hope emerged in the process of meeting others like themselves and getting to know more about this kinship. Story-telling by group members was a powerful vehicle for being exposed to and bearing witness to other's lived experience. There was a mutual understanding amongst group members that there is no greater honor that they could give one another than their rapt attention. This was part of 12-Step group process. The interactive process of telling one's story and other's attentively listening to it was recognized as having value for learning "lessons," hearing "unheard voices," and acknowledging personal "truths." It was believed that by sharing stories there lay a message that might point one in a new, better direction. It was hope-instilling to share stories of struggle and "getting better." Participants often described nearly dying because of medical complications related to their eating disorder or hitting "bottom" before joining the group. The discovery of other women who could "tell my story" was a unique, hopeful "turning point" for recovery.

> "And um, when I did go to that first meeting I felt such love and acceptance and support. And I mean, people were telling my story. People I had never met before…And, so that just kept me going back…'Cause I never found anyone who really knew what I was going through before. And that-that's what kept me there…I know at first it was, it was out of desperation [that I chose to attend]. And, I saw people getting better. I saw people who could have joy in their lives and who weren't throwing up and weren't starving. You know, were OK with

> their bodies. And so, it gave me so much hope that if I did what they had done, I too, would get better." [Participant 3, "Rose"]

"A Place to Come Together"

Hope surfaced from experiencing the group as a "safe space and place." As a haven, it allowed for self-revelation and speaking openly about one's innermost thoughts, feelings, and/or behaviors without fear of guilt, shame, stigma, or rejection. Participants often joined the group feeling imprisoned and "possessed" by the eating disorder, and, thus, walled off to others. The safety of the group space allowed them to trust the process of emotionally exploring their inner world. Women often described how they felt silenced, with no place allowing for self-expression. The group's underlying code of conduct of holding space, showing respect and non-judgment, and witnessing each other's pain and suffering, was essential for building trust. Developing trust in the 12-Step group process allowed participants to feel emotionally safe and comfortable in self-disclosure. Identifying and feeling or "sitting" with a range of emotions pushed them into new territory. In trusting one could open up so others (and self) could see "inside" inspired a fledgling hope.

> "And um, what I find today is that it's such a joy to be there. Um, it's a-it's a place where I can share my pain. A place where I can share my joy. And it's really important for me to go today to share with a newcomer, that it was like, what happened, what it's like now. Um, you know, to try and bring some hope to them, that they can get better. And it's crucial to my recovery that I continue to go to meetings...Hm, I think, oh gosh, I think the most important thing about the group is a place to come together. It's that, it's that connection that gives more hope." [Participant 3, "Rose"]

Stage 2: Sustaining Hope, Receiving Support

The second stage reflects participant's experience of germinating hope by giving and *receiving support* in ways deepening the emotional intimacy between group members and creating an atmosphere for *sustaining hope*. Hope was maintained when participants recognized how relatable other women's stories of struggling with an eating disorder were to their own story, enabling them to relate as equals and as trustworthy companions on a path to recovery.

In this stage, hope was sustained by the 12-Step program focus on fellowship and "tools." These "tools" included attending 12-Step meetings, reading 12-Step literature, e.g., the "Big Book," applying the 12-Steps and Traditions, e.g., adhering to a food plan of eating three meals and snacks per day, having a sponsor, giving service, making outreach phone calls or visits to group members, taking time for prayer and meditation, and use of the serenity prayer as a group and as individuals. The spiritual aspect of the 12-Step program, notably having faith and belief in a Higher Power (e.g., God), was a conduit for "spiritual awakening" and, in turn, "sobriety" for participants. Women stated that the spiritual aspect of the group helped create a sense of hope and healing holistically—something that was missing in their earlier encounters with traditional medical treatments. In the words of one participant:

> "I guess, you know, because I see people in the group getting better, and I, and I know myself that through working the 12 Steps I'm getting better. You know, I really put my faith in the program and in my Higher Power, and that brings me hope that I, too, will achieve what some of the others have." [Participant 3, "Rose"]

Stage 2 core-themes of the hoping process are outlined below.

"They Could Relate To the Struggle"

Hope was enhanced with participant's coming to a fuller awareness of others and their own role in the 12-Step group format, and the power of these combined roles. Group members played an active role (e.g., facilitator/leader) or a passive role (e.g., newcomer/follower), with each role being important. Group members also served as coaches (sponsors/mentors) or cheerleaders (sponsees/mentees). These roles culminated in a grouped effort moving towards change. This was about "working the Steps" together. There was a newfound awareness of accepting and understanding their eating disorder as a common struggle that tied them together, something they all struggled with. This furthered participant's ability to see recovery as possible for others and themselves—for all. Collectively unpacking and relating to the experience of what it means to "struggle" with an eating disorder, e.g., relapse in "sobriety," gave rise to hope.

> "I enjoyed going [to the self-help group with time] because people understood what I was saying. People knew how hard it was. People weren't telling me 'Well just – well, just eat, well just don't throw up.' You know, that I was getting from a lot of other aspects in my life. Um…They could relate to the struggle, and they, they loved me and accepted me even though I was really sick at the time. And cared about me…So, I know that was really important in the beginning." [Participant 3, "Rose"]

"We're All Equals"

Hope was cultivated when participants' early connections grew into well-established, mutually beneficial relationships founded on 12-Step principles and values such as honesty, equality, reciprocity, and mutuality. As "trusted servants" with no governance than a Higher Power, group members felt inherent worth and value by their very presence. This was important since feeling worthless, ineffective, inadequate, unvalued, or invisible was part of the eating disorder. They were working together in "weathering the storm" of the eating disorder and trying to "survive" it. As "helpers," participants described the importance of this equal partnership: a give-and-take style of mutual aid, support, and guidance. Reciprocity was useful if one was in a downward spiral and needed lifting up; it fed one's hope that one day she, too, would give back the same way. Group members who had maintained "sobriety" were seen as role models, not experts. Likewise, they were seen as having an equal standing, not superior to members with little to no "sobriety." Being equally yoked in 12-Step work anchored the growth of interconnection and hope.

> "You know, it's like, it's like completely mutual. The equality is really important. The fact that all of us are in the same boat. We may be at different stages of our recovery. Some of us may have a few more 24 hours [of sobriety] than others, but, we're all in the same boat. So, and uh, that's vital. That there's nobody who's an expert. There's nobody who's telling us what to do. Or, or anything like that. It's like we're all equals. We're all just bumbling along in our paths of recovery. We're just sharing what we have learned with each other and what we are learning from each other. And, we learn through one another. That's important." [Participant 7, "Janet"]

"In the Right Atmosphere Growth Happens"

Hope germinated in the group's warm social climate of trust in the 12-Step fellowship. By fellowshipping, participants sensed their own ability to trust interactions with other members and how their individual differences and uniqueness lent to the group's power to foster personal transformation. They faced growth-enhancing challenges through group interactions. For example, being challenged in one's thinking, and hence, more "sober" by perspective-taking or reality-testing. Participants acquired a richer, deeper learning of the 12-Steps, which, in turn, yielded benefits of more self-awareness, self-trust, and hope in navigating their recovery.

> "Whatever that is, um, but that honors that they carry within them the seeds of their recovery (thumps chest with hand). That, that in the right atmosphere growth happens. I see the support group as soil if we want to use that analogy. I see the support group as a, as a, uh, um, flowerbed or vegetable [garden]. It, it's got the potential, but it needs fertilizer. It needs a good digging up. It needs a recognition that not everybody's going to grow onions, but that everybody needs carrots and peas, and that pansies are just as beautiful as roses, and you know, that there's room for everybody. And I think that's important." [Participant 2, "Beth"]

Stage 3: Sharing Hope, Retelling the Story

The third stage reflects participant's experience of transplanting hope that grew from the group's essential "nutrients"—its 12-Step program philosophy, processes, and "tools"—into their lives. By sharing their lived experience, participants more fully accepted and understood their "true" self-identity, bonding as a "sisterhood," and expressing this with self-trust and self-empowerment. Participants described how *retelling the story* was an act of *sharing hope*. They embodied this hopefulness by becoming living models of hope.

In this stage, hope branched out beyond the group and into the larger community. Participant's strong desire to help other eating disordered women led to picturing a future that included sharing a "message of hope" in a public forum, thereby re-planting hope. Nearly all participants envisioned "being of service to others." A few participants had already brought this vision to life, through eating disorders awareness/activism, such as publicly speaking as recovering "addicts." Altogether, women described the 12-Step principle of "walking the talk" as a road to self-empowerment and embodiment of hope. For these women, there *was* recovery through giving testimonials on how they survived their ordeal and are now *living hope*. One participant put this into words, saying:

> "Yeah. Self-empowerment in the way where, in the way that that I've recovered from bulimia. Um, being an inspiration to other people. Um, having the guts to go like, there's this one thing I really do want to do when I, when I've recovered up, I recover. Is that, I-I do want to go give speeches. I do want to go and tell other people about it. You know, go to school[s], go to wherever need be. I'll go and talk about it. And not feel embarrassed about it because I'm living proof that it can be done." [Participant 6, "Ashley"]

Stage 3 core-themes of the hoping process are outlined below.

"I'm Just Being Me"

Hope grew as an expression of women's greater self-acceptance and self-understanding in their recovery. Participants described how the group's shared knowingness drew them closer to their own selfhood and self-knowing. Greater intimacy with oneself involved reintegrating parts of one's real, "true" self, reinventing a new one, or reclaiming a lost one—a more hopeful self. Over time, they came away feeling strengthened in their resolve to stay "sober." This also prompted a repositioning of self-identity. Participants had a stronger conviction of an inherent worth and value that surpassed societal norms for bodily beauty. This reflected admitting to others, to a Higher Power, and to themselves, flaws or defects of character per the 12-Steps. Participants focused on the reality of the body *as it is* and simply being *who they are*. This shift was pivotal for developing of a positive body image and self-image projecting a hopeful outlook.

> "I-I am still me and that that's just the way I am. You know. So I, um, that gives me hope that: I don't have to change. I don't have to change like I thought I was going to have to change? That changing isn't so much changing into another person, it's just changing my thinking about it in terms of how I think I'm supposed to act around other people (laughs), that really, I'm just being me. And, um, that gives me hope, I guess." [Participant 1, "Michelle"]

"Strong Bond with Women"

Hope thrived in deepening the emotional bonds of 12-Step fellowship. Participants described these bonds as special, treasured connections. This emotional depth and intimacy was previously lacking in their relationships with family members, friends, or clinicians. For participants, offering their story to someone else, especially a newcomer, was like re-sowing seeds of hope. For *all* sufferers, it carried the message of the 12-Steps and hope for recovery. They believed that to go forward, one has to come back to where she began, revisiting this lived experience again and again.

Retelling the story was a powerful vehicle for change. Participants acknowledged *all* group members benefited from retelling the story as a way to move forward in recovery, offering hope through a strong sense of belonging and "common welfare" as women.

> "I really feel such a strong sense of um, such a bond with women with this eating disorder. And I remember saying to myself that if I got better, this is what I want to do, is that I want to help other people. And I remember that being so strong, so...There's hope in being able to do that." [Participant 5, "Margaret"]

"To Reach Out and Let People In"

Hope flourished with participant's increased capacity for trusting and being honest with themselves, thereby embracing the whole self—body, mind, and spirit. Trusting in the will and care of a Higher Power to better their life. Trusting their real, "true" self instead of the eating disordered self. Trusting their intuition and inner wisdom. Trusting they were more sure-footed on their path to "sobriety" on account of applying the 12-Steps, which included the premise of "surrendering to their food" and the body's natural size. With more self-trust and self-honesty came more openness and willingness to risk vulnerability. For women, trusting the real, "true" self-help them to break down the inner barriers of the eating disordered self by allowing others to reach in without closing themselves off. Put another way, the hand that reached out for help became the hand that others reached in to hold for help, creating a circle of support based on trust and honesty. Expressing self-trust was needed for recovery and the blossoming of hope.

> "Just more able to give and receive love...To reach out and let people reach in. Become vulnerable and let people get to know me enough. Beginning to sort of break down some of the walls, those barriers I've had for a long time." [Participant 5, "Margaret"]

DISCUSSION

This qualitative study explored women's experience of hope in a 12-Step self-help group for eating disorders. As aforementioned, AN and BN women in this group experienced hope as a three-stage, process-oriented model with three underlying core-themes that encouraged personal change and growth over time. Participants described hope as enhancing their recovery or "sobriety," and, in fact, moving it forward. This description fits with brief descriptions of the importance of hope for recovery found in the literature (Arthur-Cameselle & Baltzell, 2012; Dawson et al., 2014; Hannon et al., 2017; Hay & Cho, 2013; Higginson & Mansell, 2008; Ibrahim & Tchanturia, 2018; Las Hayas et al., 2016; Wright & Hacking, 2012). Further, the model of hope that was revealed by studying this group suggests that hoping as a process can be accessed and re-accessed cyclically over the course of recovery. "Hoping" is a dynamic process that parallels recovery. Indeed, recovery has been described in the literature as a cyclic process (D'Abundo & Chally, 2004). An important insight gained from studying this group was that hope is a dynamic, evolving experience; it is not a static, standalone experience. Only one other study by Boisvert (2003) has articulated the paralleling of hope and recovery processes.

Participant's descriptions conveyed a strong relational component—a relational hope—embedded in each stage in the model of hope. This reflects the presence in this group of the affiliative dimension in Herth's (1991) hope model and, methodologically, van Manen's (1997) "relationality" theme. Hope requires social relationships, affirming that the group process "working" towards recovery results in the instillation of hope (Farran et al., 1995; Yalom, 2005). In this study, the model of hope presents hope from its original instillation, its ongoing maintenance by the group, and through to its projection beyond the group itself. This is a novel finding, showing that hope exists beyond its initial instillation; for eating disordered women hope is needed beyond the starting point or early phases of recovery. The OA and recovery literatures mention the "instillation of hope" as important for recovery, but do not reference hope as a necessary maintenance factor. Nor do they reference hope as relational in terms of precisely *how* hope is instilled by others. As an example, Las Hayas et al., (2016) state that in their study: "Participants also stressed the importance of the ED patient having faith and hope that recovery was possible. If they did not have this faith or hope within themselves, then it was important to have someone around them instill it in them" (pp. 586-587). Women in the ABA 12-Step self-help group clearly emphasized the need for hope as ongoing throughout their group participation; it was not a one-time injection. One other study by Herrestad and Biong (2010) similarly highlighted "relational hopes" and maintenance of hope as important for reducing self-harm behavior, particularly suicide attempts. In their study, interviews with non-eating disordered psychiatric patients (N = 12) revealed hope was relational, with three themes: (1) hopes for life, (2) hopes for death, and (3) the act of hoping. While Herrestad and Biong (2010)'s findings identify social relations as maintaining hope, and in turn, self-worth, life meaning, and preventing hopelessness that might lead to suicide, their findings do not closely explore *what* aspects of relationships infuse hope.

Women in this study described their experience of hope as intertwined with 12-Step philosophy, processes, and "tools." That is, women reported benefitting from the personal, emotional, social, and spiritual growth that corresponded with hope. It is possible the hoping process and its core-themes of accepting and understanding, connecting, and trusting represent mechanisms of change, notably 12-Step spiritual foundation, fellowship, and "tools" that can enhance recovery or "sobriety." This interpretation is akin to what has been found in OA studies, with OA members reporting OA was effective due to its spiritual and social aspects and "tools" (Hertz et al., 2012; Ronel & Libman, 2003; Russell-Mayhew et al., 2010; von Ranson et al., 2011; Wasson & Jackson, 2004). It is also on par with 12-Step literature on how the 12-Step program works, that is, its mechanisms of change, and its effectiveness in changing behavioral issues (Galanter, 2007; Khantzian & Mack, 1994).

Participants defined hope as a feeling of inner peace, tranquility, and serenity tied to a vision of a better life—a healthier life that was free of the "insanity" or "obsession" of eating disordered behaviors. This description reflects hope as goal-oriented, i.e., "I'm not going to die," and the 12-Step program's aim to better one's life and feel more serenity (Green et al., 1998; Miller, 1998). It also compliments other qualitative research suggesting recovered eating disordered women's "living in the here and now," and desire for a "new, better future without the illness" and "meaning in life" can offer motivation for living (Las Hayas et al., 2016, p. 587).

Participant's experiences that led to their finding hope in Stage 1, notably removing the stigma of the eating disorder by understanding it as an "addiction," feeling newfound acceptance for who they are as a person, i.e., their humanness as an "addict" and personal "truths," and experiencing the ABA 12-Step self-help group as an emotionally safe, secure environment, is similar to what OA members report (Hertz et al., 2012; Ronel & Libman, 2003; Russell-Mayhew et al., 2010; Wasson & Jackson, 2004).

Participant's experiences that enabled hope to be maintained in Stage 2, notably receiving support from the 12-Step program and benefit from its spiritual aspect, especially trusting in the will of a Higher Power, in the equality and reciprocity of the fellowship, and its "tools," e.g., reflecting, shifting thinking, and deepening one's learning and applying of the 12-Steps. This is akin to what has been found in OA studies (Hertz et al., 2012; Ronel & Libman, 2003; Russell-Mayhew et al., 2010; Wasson & Jackson, 2004). It also compliments Boisvert and Harrell's (2016b) finding that the spiritual benefits along with social ties enhanced the effectiveness of an ABA 12-Step treatment program. In other qualitative studies, too, the experience of "eating disorders as an in-group" and "collective identification" in general (non-12-Step-oriented) eating disorder support groups has been identified as helpful for recovery (Ison & Kent, 2010; Powers Koski, 2014).

Participant's experiences culminated in projecting hope in Stage 3, re-telling their story and "being of service to others" by carrying the message of the 12-Steps and its role in fostering their hope, establishing a healthier, hopeful self-identity, and having self-honesty and self-trust in recovery. This is similar to what is reported by Boisvert (2003) and OA studies (Russell-Mayhew et al., 2010).

Trust as a core-theme of hope is an interesting finding from this study, and is important for clinical practice (see below). Previous research by Boisvert (2001) found a relationship between lower hope and greater eating disorder symptom severity in AN and BN women, particularly interpersonal distrust and social insecurity. Perhaps this unique finding is a function of the study sample, reflecting the strength of participant's trust in the 12-Step program, with "trusting" having meaning in terms of being "honest" with others and oneself about the reality of their illness severity, or being taken care of by others taking care of self. While the present study offers a glimpse into the importance of trusting for hope, the meaning of trust from the perspective of eating disordered women in 12-Step groups requires further exploration.

Finally, the present study suggests that group interaction can be powerful for women's development of hopefulness as well as their self-development, self-empowerment, and self-transformation. A subtle finding was that hope intersected with becoming known to others and oneself, that is, acquiring more self-knowledge through relationships in the 12-Step group, including with a Higher Power, e.g., God. It may be that in feeling a sense of belonging in a "common welfare" as a "sisterhood," women's relational "way of knowing" (Belenky et al., 1997) was honored and brought to the fore of the group, facilitating agency, self-empowerment, and personal growth. This finding of increased self-knowing and knowingness, and creating a sense of community and connectedness in order to facilitate personal growth and recovery compliments research on women's recovery. The "development of self-awareness," "gaining self-knowledge," and self-empowerment have also been identified as themes in other qualitative studies (Duncan et al., 2015; Las Hayas et al., 2016; Nordbø et al., 2008; Pivarunas, 2016).

LIMITATIONS AND FUTURE DIRECTIONS

This study explored a novel topic. This strength allows this study to make a unique, valuable contribution to the literature and further inroads in research. Participants' descriptions of 12-Step group processes provided insight into the meaning of hope, that is, to feel acceptance and understanding, connecting, and trusting in a way that enhances recovery. The experience of hope as a dynamic, evolving process and its core-themes requires additional data to confirm if, in fact, it is a determinant of change, with the potential to move women forward in recovery.

Data collection using observation and interviews are methodological strengths. The stories of the women in this study were heartfelt and honest; providing tremendous insight into the struggle of having an eating disorder while also having hope for a life freed of it. The researcher's up-close, subjective perspective of group interactions and processes yielded insights into and an understanding of participant's experiences about hoping. These could not have been acquired from an arms-length, objective perspective or methodology, such as a one-time survey.

Despite these strengths, several limitations need to be mentioned. First, there was a deliberate focus on eating disordered women in a 12-Step self-help group in the community. Thus, this was a self-selected group. This was a convenience sample. Therefore, results need to be interpreted in terms of possible selection bias, recognizing that they cannot necessarily be generalized to other self-help groups. It is possible that women attending other 12-Step self-help groups for eating disorders, e.g., OA, or addictions to alcohol and/or drugs, e.g., Alcoholics Anonymous (AA), Narcotics Anonymous (NA), might differ in their experience of hope.

Second, because group membership was comprised of women at the time of the study, no data were collected on men. Eating disordered men with similar characteristics and/or involvement in 12-Step self-help groups could be interviewed. Similarly, other eating disordered individuals with diverse characteristics could be studied. Exploring gender and diversity issues, e.g., sizeism, when treating eating disorders is important (Boisvert, 2012b). Future research should consider how these issues might influence a patient's experience of hope in clinical work.

Third, only self-report data on eating disorder diagnosis were collected. Research has shown that the overarching diagnostic category of "eating disorder" is stable (Milos et al., 2005). However, there is considerable "diagnostic flux within the eating disorders" (Milos et al., 2005, p. 573). Eating disorder subtypes, symptom severity, or chronicity might adversely affect patients by lowering their hope, making it difficult for them to contemplate change, comply with traditional treatments, or plan for a future that entails a better quality of life. Clearly, more data is needed on specific aspects of eating disorders in relation to hopefulness.

Fourth, participants reported the benefits of group participation, including 12-Step philosophy, processes, and "tools," in fostering hope and recovery. However, participants' subjective reflections should not be construed as an objective evaluation of the effectiveness of 12-Step groups for treating eating disorders.

Implications for Practice

For participants, hope was a process grounded in the relational aspect of the 12-Step self-help group. This subjective knowledge must be recognized and incorporated into clinical practice. Practitioners need to clearly understand the clinical utility of hope when treating eating disordered patients, especially it being instrumental for helping these patients move towards recovery. The model of hope that was revealed in this study provides practitioners with a resource to guide their interactions and tailor interventions to increase hope in their patients. This is important when one considers that therapeutic alliance is based on themes of acceptance and understanding, connecting, and trusting. A strong therapeutic alliance reflecting trust and empathy is associated with therapeutic change and treatment effectiveness (Wampold, 2015). The use of hope-focused interventions, (i.e., using the word hope or hop*ing*) can enhance therapeutic alliance, change process, and hope (Larsen & Stege, 2010a, 2010b).

Eating disorder patients find psychological interventions, i.e., talk therapy, to be helpful, especially when professional relationships are experienced as caring, empathic, and supportive (Akey et al., 2013; Akey & Rintamaki, 2014; Cockell et al., 2004; de la Rie et al., 2006; Linville et al., 2012; Pettersen & Rosenvinge, 2002; Rich, 2006; for reviews, see Bell, 2003; Bezance & Holliday, 2013; Wetzler et al., 2020). Evans et al. (2011) studied and found that for bulimic-type eating disordered women: "Empathy, providing information and hope were considered important features of health professionals" (p. 271). Practitioners can also be helpful to these patients by evaluating and exploring their hope as an act of hoping and as a meaningful act of living.

Practitioners should consider evaluating patient's level of hope using Herth's (1991, 1992) hope scales/indices. And, if patients report lowered hope, i.e., hopelessness, then also assessing for suicidality per the three-step theory (3ST) outlined by Klonsky and May (2015). This might provide an indication of patient's hopelessness, social disconnection, or possible need for self-harm reduction or suicide prevention. Patient's responses to particular measure items can be an opportunity to talk about a need for more hope and how to access this inner resource.

A strategy for increasing hope can include encouraging patients to identify positive life experiences, memories, persons, or connections that can cultivate their hope (Boisvert, 2003). Another strategy is patient's making a "hope box" filled with objects, e.g., personal mementoes, letters, pictures, that they can access when they feel hopeless. This can be an actual box or a virtual box, e.g., patients putting pictures into their cell phone or other digital device(s). Yet another strategy involves writing prompts or exercises designed to tap hope such as: Who made you feel accepted or understood so that you felt some hope today? What did you do today to feel connected to self/others in a way(s) that felt hopeful to you? Was there an opportunity today for you to trust someone in a way(s) that gave you hope?

Practitioners can also use cognitive-behavioral (CBT) or dialectical-behavioral therapy (DBT) interventions to help increase patient's hope by shifting a viewpoint or cultivating meaning in life experiences (Fairburn, 2008; Safer et al., 2017). CBT and DBT would seem to be promising treatment modalities for low-hope eating disordered women since hope provides a person with a cognitive framework and belief that "life is worth living." Inversely, helping patients create a "life worth living" may increase hope. To be effective, a practitioner should consider applying CBT and DBT interventions to less hopeful patients in order to develop a repertoire of successive, attainable steps or "goals" for altering eating disordered behaviors. In other words, practitioners should role model, "teach," and reinforce behavior that mimics that of healthy, hopeful women.

In addition to professional support, speaking with another eating disorder sufferer is a critical factor in eating disordered women's recovery (Beveridge et al., 2019; Cockell et al., 2004; Nicholls et al., 2016). This study found eating disordered women's need for mutual support from other women who can "relate to the struggle" or are also "telling my story" was intimately tied to their experiencing of hope. Practitioners need to understand how 12-Step programs work and how they can augment CBT interventions, e.g., cognitive restructuring, and DBT interventions, e.g., sitting with emotions (Fairburn, 2008; Safer et al., 2017; Steigerwald & Stone, 1999). Practitioners should provide referrals for 12-Step (or other self-help) groups that might offer a safe, supportive environment in which women can feel comfortable sharing their personal stories and wherein hope can become embedded into their stories. Indeed, practitioners often report referring their eating disordered patients to 12-Step self-help groups in the community, e.g., OA, for adjunct treatment (von Ranson et al., 2013). These referrals are crucial when practitioners understand eating disordered women's hope arises, grows, and branches out of relationships with others in these groups, uniting them in overcoming an "addiction."

The spiritual foundation of 12-Step self-help groups for eating disorders may be adapted to the clinical setting (Boisvert & Harrell,

2016b; Johnson & Sansone, 1993; Johnson & Taylor, 1996; Yeary, 1987). Like hope, spirituality has relevance for eating disorders (Boisvert & Harrell, 2013a, 2013b, 2016a). Further research on the spiritual benefits of 12-Step groups in clinical and community settings can establish their effectiveness for increasing hope and, in turn, treating eating disorders. Practitioners might tie into treatment specific spiritual or "faith" elements to promote hope and connectedness, including a Higher Power, e.g., God, while remaining respectful of patient's beliefs (Pivarunas, 2016). This might increase patient's sense of belonging and "wholeness," as well as integration of a hopeful self-identity and spirituality.

Practitioners might also use adjuncts in unconventional, innovative ways that give "voice" to women's experiences of hope and recovery—either verbally through metaphoric language, or nonverbally through photography (Boisvert, 2003, 2012a; Mathieson & Hoskins, 2005). Indeed, a few of the women used metaphor when describing their hope or the 12-Step self-help group. For example, Participant 5, "Margaret," described hope as "The light at the other side—the other end of the tunnel, you know." As another example, Participant 3, "Beth" described the self-help group as a "flowerbed or vegetable [garden]." As a last example, Participant 7, "Janet," described the humanness and togetherness of 12-Step recovery work, stating, "…we're all in the same boat…We're all just bumbling along in our paths of recovery." Acutely ill AN or BN women might have difficulty identifying or feeling their emotions or putting their experiences into words, i.e., alexithymic. Such was the case with Participant 4, "Marie," who was acutely ill and described, "It's really, really hard for me to picture it," when asked to put into words an image of hope. In these instances, the use of visual media such as art or photography might be helpful by providing patients a means for exploring and expressing their inner worlds nonverbally with pictures or images, and to feel emotionally safer using this form of self-exploration and self-expression. Practitioners are encouraged to use these adjuncts to tap patient's experiences of hope and recovery processes.

Summary and Conclusion

This exploratory qualitative study offers insight into seven eating disordered women's experience of hope in a 12-Step self-help group. The women described hope as a process of finding, maintaining, and projecting hope emerging from three core-themes of accepting and understanding, connecting, and trusting. The process-oriented model of hope adds a vital, new dimension to the research literature on eating disorders in women, requiring further investigation.

This study points to the potential to delve further into the experience of hope for eating disordered women who are at various stages of illness and participating in alternative treatments such as 12-Step self-help groups. Greater understanding of the meaning of hope for eating disordered women along with those specific factors in 12-Step self-help groups that give rise to hopeful experiences can inform practitioner's knowledge and use of hope-focused interventions. Practitioners should be aware of the importance of hope and apt at instilling hope in order to treat effectively this special population. Practitioners should convey a hopeful outlook for their eating disorder patients in clinical work as doing so might inspire their desire to improve, recover, and become a living image of hope.

Acknowledgments

Appreciation is extended to Ronna F. Jevne, PhD. and Cheryl L. Nekolaichuk, PhD. for their expertise in hope and qualitative research, and to The Hope Foundation of Alberta for its financial support. Appreciation is also extended to W. Andrew Harrell, PhD. for his feedback and comments. Thanks are given to the seven women who participated in this study.

References

Abbate-Daga, G., Amianto, F., Delsedime, N., De-Bacco, C., & Fassino, S. (2013). Resistance to treatment and change in anorexia nervosa: A clinical review. *BMC Psychiatry, 13*:294. doi: 10.1186/1471-244X-13-294.

Abbate-Daga, G., Facchini, F., Marzola, E., Delsedime, N., Giovannone, C., Amianto, F., & Fassino, S. (2014). Health-related quality of life in adult inpatients affected by anorexia nervosa. *European Eating Disorders Review, 22*, 285-291. doi: 10.1002/erv.2302.

Acharya, T., & Agius, M. (2017). The importance of hope against other factors in the recovery of mental illness. *Psychiatria Danubina, 29*(3), 619-622.

Alcoholics Anonymous World Services. (1939). *Alcoholics Anonymous*. New York: Author.

Alcoholics Anonymous World Services. (1952). *Twelve Steps and Twelve Traditions*. New York: Author.

Alcoholics Anonymous World Services. (1955). *Alcoholics Anonymous: The story of how many thousands of men and women have recovered from alcoholism*. New York: Author.

Akey, J. E., & Rintamaki, L. S. (2014). Optimal social support practices for health care professionals who treat patients managing eating disorders. *Journal of Nervous & Mental Disease, 202*(2), 126-132. doi:10.1097/NMD.0000000000000081.

Akey, J. E., & Rintamaki, L. S., & Kane, T. L. (2013). Health belief model deterrents of social support seeking among people coping with eating disorders. *Journal of Affective Disorders, 145*, 246-252. doi: 10.1016/j.jad.2012.04.045.

American Psychiatric Association. (2013). *Diagnostic and statistical manual of mental disorders: DSM-5* (5th ed.). Arlington, VA: Author.

Anorexics and Bulimics Anonymous. (2002). *Anorexics and Bulimics Anonymous: The fellowship details its program of recovery for anorexia and bulimia*. Edmonton, Alberta: Author.

Arcelus, J., Mitchell, A. J., Wales, J., & Nielsen, S. (2011). Mortality rates in patients with anorexia nervosa and other eating disorders: A meta-analysis of 36 studies. *Archives of General Psychiatry, 68*(7), 742-731. doi: 10.1001/archgenpsychiatry.2011.74.

Arthur-Cameselle, J.N., & Baltzell, A. (2012). Learning from collegiate athletes who have recovered from eating disorders: Advice to coaches, parents, and other athletes with eating disorders. *Journal of Applied Sport Psychology, 24*(1), 1-9. doi: 10.1080/10413200. 2011.572949.

Bell, L. (2003). What can we learn from consumer studies and qualitative research in the treatment of eating disorders? *Eating & Weight Disorders, 8*, 181-187.

Belenky, M., Clinchy, B. M., Goldberger, N. R., & Tarule, J. M. (1997). *Women's ways of knowing: The development of self, voice, and mind* (10th ed.). New York: Basic Books.

Beveridge, J., Phillipou, A., Jenkins, Z., Newton, R., Brennan, L., Hanly, F., Torrens-Witherow, B., Warren, N., Edwards, K., & Castle, D. (2019). Peer mentoring for eating disorders: results from the evaluation of a pilot program. *Journal of Eating Disorders, 7*:13, 1-10. doi: 10.1183/s40337-019-0245-3.

Bezance, J., & Holliday, J. (2013). Adolescents with anorexia nervosa have their say: A review of qualitative studies on treatment and recovery from anorexia nervosa. *European Eating Disorders Review, 21*, 352-360. doi: 10.1002/erv.2239.

Björk, T., & Ahlström, G. (2008). The patient's perception of having recovered from an eating disorder. *Health Care for Women International, 29*, 926-944. doi: 10.1080/07399330802269543.

Boisvert, J. A. (2001). *The relationship between level of hope and coping in eating disordered women*. Unpublished master's thesis. University of Regina, Regina, Saskatchewan.

Boisvert, J. A. (2003). A visual diary of an anorexic woman: Development of a hopeful self-healer identity. *Canadian Journal of Counselling, 37*(1), 28-34.

Boisvert, J. A. (2006). The relationship between hope, coping, spirituality and eating disorder symptomatology in women. *Dissertation Abstracts International: Section B: The Sciences and Engineering, 66*(9-B), 5078.

Boisvert, J. A. (2012a). Exploring self-healing: Seeing life through a new lens. In R. F. Jevne (Ed.), *Images & echoes: Exploring life with photography and writing* (pp. 141-153). Edmonton, AB: Elskie Consulting.

Boisvert, J. A. (2012b). Native American Indian women, fat studies and feminism. *Somatechnics, 2*(1), 84-92. doi: 10.3366/soma.2012.0042.

Boisvert, J. A., & Harrell, W. A. (2009a). Homosexuality as a risk factor for eating disorder symptomatology in men. *Journal of Men's Studies, 17*(3), 210-225. doi: 10.3149/jms.1703.210.

Boisvert, J. A., & Harrell, W. A. (2009b). The impact of English-speaking in the household and immigrant generational household on eating disorder symptomatology among Canadian women and men. *Women's Health & Urban Life, 8*(2), 64-83.

Boisvert, J. A., & Harrell, W. A. (2012). Ethnicity and spirituality as risk factors for eating disorder symptomatology in men. *International Journal of Men's Health*, *11*(1), 36-62. doi: 10.3149/jmh.1101.36.

Boisvert, J. A., & Harrell, W. A. (2013a). The effects of hope, body shame and body mass index on eating disorder symptomatology in women. *International Journal of Psychology Research, 8*(3), 207-226.

Boisvert, J. A., & Harrell, W. A. (2013b). The impact of spirituality on eating disorder symptomatology in ethnically diverse Canadian women. *International Journal of Social Psychiatry, 59*(8), 729-738. doi: 10.1177/0020764012453816.

Boisvert, J. A., & Harrell, W. A. (2016a). Spirituality, religiosity and eating disorder symptomatology in women. In R. Cooper (Ed.), *Religiosity: Psychological perspectives, individual differences and health benefits* (pp. 103-192). Hauppauge, NY: Nova Publishers.

Boisvert, J. A., & Harrell, W. A. (2016b). A Twelve-Step day treatment program for women with eating disorders: Examining treatment effectiveness and spiritual health benefits. In N. Morton (Ed.), *Eating disorders: Prevalence, risk factors and treatment options* (pp. 224-270). Hauppauge, NY: Nova Publishers.

Buckley, J., & Herth, K. (2004). Fostering hope in terminally ill patients. *Nursing Standard, 19*(10), 33-41.

Button, E. J., & Warren, R. L. (2001). Living with anorexia nervosa: The experience of a cohort of sufferers from anorexia nervosa 7.5 years after initial presentation to a specialized eating disorder service. *European Eating Disorders Review, 9*(2), 74-76. doi: 10.1002/erv.400.

Cockell, S. J., Zaitsoff, S. L., & Geller, J. (2004). Maintaining change following eating disorder treatment. *Professional Psychology: Research and Practice, 35*(5), 527-534. doi: 10.1037/0735-7028.35.5.527.

D'Abundo, M., & Chally, P. (2004). Struggling with recovery: Participant perspectives on battling an eating disorder. *Qualitative Health Research, 14*(8), 1094-1106. doi; 10.1177/1049732304267753.

Dawson, L., Rhodes, P., & Touyz, S. (2014). "Doing the impossible": The process of recovery from chronic anorexia nervosa. *Qualitative Health Research, 24*(4), 494-505. doi: 10.1177/1049732314524029.

de la Rie, S., Noordenbos, G., Donker, M., & van Furth, E. (2006). Evaluating the treatment of eating disorders from the patient's perspective. *International Journal of Eating Disorders, 39*, 667-676. doi: 10.1002/eat.20317.

de Vos, J. A., LaMarre, A., Radstaak, M., Bijkerk, C. A., Bohlmeijer, E. T., & Westerhof, G. J. (2017). Identifying fundamental criteria for eating disorder recovery: A systematic review and qualitative meta-analysis. *Journal of Eating Disorders, 5*:34, 1-14. doi: 10.1186/s40337-017-0164-0.

Denzin, N. K., & Lincoln, Y. S. (1998). Introduction: Entering the field of qualitative research. In N. K. Denzin & Y. S. Lincoln (Eds.), *Strategies of qualitative inquiry* (pp. 1-34). Thousand Oaks: Sage.

Denzin, N. K., & Lincoln, Y. S. (2000). Introduction: The discipline and practice of qualitative research. In N. K. Denzin & Y. S. Lincoln (Eds.), *Handbook of qualitative research* (2nd ed., pp. 1-29). Thousand Oaks: Sage.

Doe, M. J. (2019). Conceptual foreknowings: An integrative review of hope. *Nursing Science Quarterly, 33*(1), 55-64. doi: 10.1177/0894318419881805.

Duncan, T. K., Sebar, B., & Lee, J. (2015). Reclamation of power and self: A meta-synthesis exploring the process of recovery from anorexia nervosa. *Advances in Eating Disorders: Theory, Research, and Practice, 3*(2), 177-190. doi: 10.1080/21662630.2014.978804.

Espíndola, C. R., & Blay, S. L. (2009). Anorexia nervosa treatment from the patient perspective: A metasynthesis of qualitative studies. *Annals of Clinical Psychiatry, 21*(1), 38-48.

Evans, E. J., Hay, P. J., Mond, J., Paxton, S. J., Quirk, F., Rodgers, B., Jhajj, A., K., & Sawoniewska, M. A. (2011). Barriers to help-seeking in young women with eating disorders: A qualitative exploration in a longitudinal community survey. *Eating Disorders, 19*, 270-285. doi: 10.1080/10640266.2011.566152.

Fairburn, C. G. (2008). *Cognitive behavior therapy and eating disorders*. New York: Guilford.

Fairburn, C. G., & Harrison, P. J. (2003). Eating disorders. *Lancet, 361*(9355), 407-416. doi: 10.1016/S0140-6736(03)12378-1.

Farran, C. J., Herth, K. A., & Popovich, J. M. (1995). *Hope and hopelessness: Critical clinical constructs*. Newbury Park, CA: Sage.

Federici, A., & Kaplan, A. S. (2008). The patient's account of relapse and recovery in anorexia nervosa: A qualitative study. *European Eating Disorders Review, 16*, 1-10. doi: 10.1002/erv.813.

Forcano, L., Álvarez, E., Santamaria, J. J., Jimenez-Murcia, S., Granero, R., Penelo, E., Alonso, P., Sánchez, I., Menchón, J. M., Ulman, F., Bulik, C. M., & Fernández-Aranda, F. (2011). Suicide attempts in anorexia nervosa subtypes. *Comprehensive Psychiatry, 52*(4), 352-358. doi: 10.1016/j.comppsych.2010.09.003.

Franko, D. L., Keshaviah, A., Eddy, K. T., Krishna, M., Davis, M. C., Keel, P. K., & Herzog, D. B. (2013). A longitudinal investigation of mortality in anorexia nervosa and bulimia nervosa. *American Journal of Psychiatry, 170*, 917-925. doi: 10.1176/appl.ajp.2013.12070868

Galanter, M. (2007). Spirituality and recovery in 12-Step programs: An empirical model. *Journal of Substance Abuse Treatment, 33(3)*, 265-272. doi: 10.1016/j.jsat.2007.04.016.

Gordon, R. A. (2000). *Eating disorders: Anatomy of a social epidemic* (2nd ed.). Malden, MA: Wiley-Blackwell.

Green, L. L., Fullilove, M. T., & Fullilove, R. E. (1998). Stories of spiritual awakening: The nature of spirituality in recovery. *Journal of Substance Abuse Treatment, 15*(4), 325-331. doi: 10.1016/S0740-5472(97)00211-0.

Guba, E. G. (1981). Criteria for assessing the trustworthiness of naturalistic inquiries. *Educational Communication and Technology Journal, 29*(2), 75-91. doi: 10.1007/bf02766777.

Guba, E. G., & Lincoln, Y. S. (1981). *Effective evaluation: Improving the usefulness of evaluation result through responsive and naturalistic approaches*. San Francisco, CA: Jossey-Bass.

Guba, E. G., & Lincoln, Y. S. (1982). Epistemological and methodological bases of naturalistic inquiry. *Educational Communication and Technology Journal, 30*(4), 233-252.

Guillame, S., Jaussent, I., Oilié, E., Genty, C., Bringer, J., Courtet, P., & Schmidt, U. (2011). Characteristics of suicide attempts in anorexia and bulimia nervosa: A case-control study. *PLoS ONE 6*(8): e23578. doi: 10.1371/journal.pone.0023578.

Hannon, J., Eunson, L., & Munro, C. (2017). The patient experience of illness, treatment, and change, during intensive community treatment for severe anorexia nervosa. *Eating Disorders, 25*(4), 279-296. doi: 10.1080/10640266.2017.1318626.

Hay, P. J., & Cho, K. (2013). A qualitative exploration of influences on the process of recovery from personal written accounts of people with anorexia nervosa. *Women & Health, 53*(7), 730-740. doi: 10.1080/03630242.2013.821694.

Herrestad, H., & Biong, S. (2010). Relational hopes: A study of the lived experience of hope in some patients hospitalized for intentional self-harm. *International Journal of Qualitative Studies on Health and Well-Being, 5*(1), 1-9. doi: 10.3402/qhw.v5i1.4651.

Herth, K. (1987). *The relationship between level of hope and level of coping response in cancer patients.* Unpublished doctoral dissertation. Texas Woman's University, Texas.

Herth, K. (1989). The relationship between level of hope and level of coping response and other variables in patients with cancer. *Oncology Nursing Forum, 16*(1), 67-72.

Herth, K. (1990). Fostering hope in terminally-ill people. *Journal of Advanced Nursing, 15*(11), 1250-1259. doi: 10.1111/j.1365-2648.1990.tb01740.x.

Herth, K. (1991). Development and refinement of an instrument to measure hope. *Scholarly Inquiry for Nursing Practice: An International Journal, 59*(1), 39-51.

Herth, K. (1992). Abbreviated instrument to measure hope: Development and psychometric evaluation. *Journal of Advanced Nursing, 17*(10), 1251-1259. doi: 10.1111/j.1365-2648.1992.tb01843.x.

Herth, K. (1993). Hope in older adults in community and institutional settings. *Issues in Mental Health Nursing, 14*(2), 139-156. doi: 10.3109/01612849309031613.

Herth, K. (1996). Hope from the perspective of homeless families. *Journal of Advanced Nursing, 24*(4), 743-753. doi: 10.1046/j.1365-2648.1996.25113.x.

Hertz, P., Addad, M., & Ronel, N. (2012). Attachment styles and changes among women members of Overeaters Anonymous who have recovered from binge-eating disorder. *Health & Social Work, 37*(2), 110-122. doi: 10.1093/hsw/hls019.

Herzog, D. B., Greenwood, D. N., Dorer, D. J., Flores, A. T., Ekeblad, E. R., Richards, A., Blais, M. A., & Keller, M. B. (2000). Mortality in eating disorders: A descriptive study. *International Journal of Eating Disorders, 28*(1), 20-26. doi: 10.1002/(SICI)1098-108X(200007) 28;1<20::AID-EAT>3.0.C);2-X.

Hesse-Biber, S., Leavy, P., Quinn, C. E., & Zoino, J. (2006). The mass marketing of disordered eating and Eating Disorders: The social psychology of women, thinness and culture. *Women's Studies International Forum, 29*, 208-224. doi: 10.1016/j.wsif.2006.03.007.

Higginson, S., & Mansell, W. (2008). A qualitative analysis of six individuals who experienced personal change and recovery. *Psychology and Psychotherapy, 81*, 309-328. doi: 10.1348/14760 8308X320125.

Hoek, H. W. (2006). Incidence, prevalence and mortality of anorexia nervosa and other eating disorders. *Current Opinion in Psychiatry, 19*(4), 389-394. doi: 10.1097/01.yco.0000228759.95237.78.

Hoek, H. W., & van Hoeken, D. (2003). Review of the prevalence and incidence of eating disorders. *International Journal of Eating Disorders, 34*(4), 383-396. doi: 10.1002/eat.10222.

Hsu, L. K. G., Crisp, A. H., & Callender, J. S. (1992). Recovery in anorexia nervosa –The patient's perspective. *International Journal of Eating Disorders, 11*(4), 341-350. doi: 10.1002/1098-108X (199205)11:4<341::AID-EAT2260110408>3.0.CO;2-G.

Hudson, J. I., Hiripi, E., Pope, H. G., Jr., & Kessler, R. C. (2007). The prevalence and correlates of eating disorders in the National Comorbidity Survey Replication. *Biological Psychiatry, 61*(3), 348-358. doi: 10.1016/j.biopsych.2006.03.040.

Huen, M. Y., Ip, B. Y., Ho, S. M. Y., & Yip, P. S. F. (2015). Hope and hopelessness: The role of hope in buffering the impact of hopelessness on suicidal ideation. *PLoS ONE 10*(6): e0130073. doi: 10.1371/journal.pone.0130073.

Ison, J., & Kent, S. (2010). Social identity in eating disorders. *European Eating Disorders Review, 18*, 475-485. doi: 10.1002/erv.1001.

Jenkins, J., & Ogden, J. (2012). Becoming "whole" again: A qualitative study of women's views of recovering from anorexia nervosa. *European Eating Disorders Review, 20*(1), e23-e31. doi: 10.1002/erv.1085.

Johnson, C. L., & Sansone, R. A. (1993). Integrating the Twelve-Step approach with traditional psychotherapy for the treatment of eating disorders. *International Journal of Eating Disorders, 14*(2), 121-134. doi: 10.1002/1098-108X(199309)14:2<2121::AID-EAT22601402 02.3.CO;2-N.

Johnson, C. L., & Taylor, C. (1996). Working with difficult-to-treat eating disorders using an integration of Twelve-Step and traditional psychotherapies. *Psychiatric Clinics of North America, 19*(4), 829-841. doi: 10.1016/S0193-953X(05)70384-1.

Klein, D. A., & Walsh, B. T. (2004). Eating disorders: Clinical features and pathophysiology. *Physiology & Behavior, 81*(2), 359-374. doi: 10.1016/j.physbeh.2004.02.009.

Klonsky, E. D., & May, A. M. (2015). The Three-Step Theory (3ST): A new theory of suicide rooted in the "ideation-to-action" framework. *International Journal of Cognitive Therapy 8(2)*, 114-129. doi: 10.1521/ijct.2015.8.2.114.

Larsen, D. J., & Stege, R. (2010a). Hope-focused practices during early psychotherapy sessions. Part 1: Implicit approaches. *Journal of Psychotherapy Integration, 20*(3), 271-292. doi: 10.1037/a0020820.

Larsen, D. J., & Stege, R. (2010b). Hope-focused practices during early psychotherapy sessions. Part 2: Explicit approaches. *Journal of Psychotherapy Integration, 20*(3), 293-311. doi: 10.1037/a0020821.

Las Hayas, C., Padierna, J. A., Muñoz, P., Aguirre, M., Gómez del Barrio, A., Beato-Fernández, L., & Calvete, E. (2016). Resilience in eating disorders: A qualitative study. *Women & Health, 56*(5), 576-594. doi: 10.1080/03630242.2015.1101744.

Lewinsohn, P. M., Seeley, J. R., Moerk, K. C., & Striegel-Moore, R. H. (2002). Gender differences in eating disorder symptoms in young adults. *International Journal of Eating Disorders, 32*, 426-440. doi: 10.1002/eat.10103.

Lincoln, Y. S., & Guba, E. G. (2000). Paradigmic controversies, contractions, and emerging confluences. In N. K. Denzin & Y. S. Lincoln (Eds.), *Handbook of qualitative research* (2nd ed., pp. 163-188). Thousand Oaks, CA: Sage.

Lindgren, B-M., Enmark, A., Bohman, A., & Lundström, M. (2015). A qualitative study of young women's experiences of recovery from bulimia nervosa. *Journal of Advanced Nursing, 71*(4), 860-869. doi: 10.1111/jan.12554.

Linville, D., Brown, T., Sturm, K., & McDougal, T. (2012). Eating disorders and social support: Perspectives of recovered individuals. *Journal of Treatment & Prevention, 20*(3), 216-231. doi: 10.1080/10640266.668480.

Mathieson, L. C., & Hoskins, M. L. (2005). Metaphors of change in the context of eating disorders: Bridging understanding with girls' perceptions. *Canadian Journal of Counseling, 39*(4), 260-274.

Milos, G., Spindler, A., Schnyder, U., & Fairburn, C. G. (2005). Instability of eating disorder diagnoses: Prospective study. *British Journal of Psychiatry, 187*(6), 573-578. doi: 10.1192/bjp.197.6.573.

Miller, W. R. (1998). Researching the spiritual dimensions of alcohol and other drug problems. *Addiction, 93*(7), 979-990. doi: 10.1046/j.1360-0443.1998.937979.x.

Morse, J. M., & Doberneck, B. M. (1995). Delineating the concept of hope. *IMAGE: Journal of Nursing Scholarship, 27*(4), 277-285. doi: 10.1111/j.1547-50691995.tb00888.x.

Morse, J. M., & Field, P. A. (1995). *Qualitative research methods for health professionals* (2nd ed.). Thousand Oaks, CA: Sage.

Morse, J. M., & Penrod, J. (1999). Linking concepts of enduring, uncertainty, suffering, and hope. *IMAGE: Journal of Nursing Scholarship, 31*(2), 145-150. doi: 10.1111/j.1547-5069.1999.tb0 455.x.

Murnen, S. K., & Smolak, L. (2015). Gender and eating disorders. In L. Smolak & M. P. Levine (Eds.), *The Wiley handbook of eating disorders* (Vol. 1, pp. 352-366). Sussex, England: Wiley.

Nekolaichuk, C. L. (1995). *An exploration of the meaning of hope in health and illness*. Unpublished doctoral dissertation. University of Alberta, Edmonton, Alberta.

Nekolaichuk, C. L., & Bruera, E. (1998). On the nature of hope in palliative care. *Journal of Palliative Care, 14*(1), 36-42. doi: 10.1177/082585979801400107.

Nekolaichuk, C. L., Jevne, R. F., & Maguire, T. O. (1999). Structuring the meaning of hope in health and illness. *Social Science & Medicine, 48*(5), 591-605. doi: 10.1016/S0277-9536(98)00348-7.

Nicholls, D., Fogarty, S., Hay, P., & Ramjan, L. (2016). Participatory action research for women with anorexia nervosa. *Nurse Researcher, 23*(5), 26-30. doi: 10.7748/nr.23.5.26.s6.

Noordenbos, G. (1989). Improving the process of recovery of patients with anorexia nervosa. *British Review of Bulimia & Anorexia Nervosa, 3*(1), 17-32.

Noordenbos, G., Jacobs, M. E., & Hertzberger, E. (1998). Chronic eating disorders: The patients' view of their treatment history. *Eating Disorders, 6*(3), 7-13. doi: 10.1080/10640269808249256.

Nordbø, R. H. S., Gulliksen, K. S., Espeset, E. M. S., Skårderud, F., Geller, J., & Holte, A. (2008). Expanding the concept of motivation to change: The content of patients' wish to recover from anorexia nervosa. *International Journal of Eating Disorders, 41*, 635-642. doi: 10.1002/eat.20547.

Patton, M. Q. (2002). *Qualitative evaluation and research methods* (3rd ed.). Newbury Park, CA: Sage.

Petterson, G., & Rosenvinge, J. H. (2002). Improvement and recovery from eating disorders: A patient perspective. *Journal of Treatment & Prevention, 10*(1), 61-71.

Pivarunas, B. (2016). A qualitative exploration of a faith-based support group for women with disordered eating. *Pastoral Psychology, 65*, 215-225. doi: 10.1007/s11089-015-0675-z.

Powers Koski, J. (2014). "I'm just a walking eating disorder": The mobilisation and construction of a collective illness identity in eating disorder support groups. *Sociology of Health & Illness, 36*(1), 75-90. doi: 10.1111/1467-9566.12044.

Reinharz, S. (1992). *Feminist methods in social research*. New York: Oxford University Press.

Rich, E. (2006). Anorexic dis(connection): Managing anorexia as an illness and an identity. *Sociology of Health & Illness, 28*(3), 284-305. doi: 10.1111/j.1467-9566.2006.00493.x.

Rome, E. S., & Ammerman, S. (2003). Medical complications of eating disorders: An update. *Journal of Adolescent Health, 33*(6), 418-426. doi:10.1016/j.jadohealth.2003.07.002.

Ronel, N., & Libman, G. (2003). Eating disorders and recovery: Lessons from Overeaters Anonymous. *Clinical Social Work Journal, 31*, 155-171.

Rorty, M., Yager, J., & Rossotto, E. (1993). Why and how do women recover from bulimia nervosa? The subjective appraisals of forty women recovered for a year or more. *International Journal of Eating Disorders, 14*(3), 249-260. doi: 10.1002/1098-108(199311)14:3 <249::AID-EAT226014030>3.0.CO;2-O.

Russell-Mayhew, S., von Ranson, K. M., & Masson, P. C. (2010). How does Overeaters Anonymous help its members? A qualitative analysis. *European Eating Disorders Review, 18*, 33-42. doi: 10.1002/erv.966.

Safer, D. L., Telch, C. F., & Chen, E. Y. (2017). *Dialectical behavior therapy for binge eating and bulimia*. New York: Guilford.

Smolak, L., & Murnen, S. K. (2001). Gender and eating problems. In R. H. Striegel-Moore & L. Smolak (Eds.), *Eating disorders: Innovative directions in research and practice (Vol. 1): Basic concepts and foundational research* (pp. 91-110). Washington, DC: American Psychological Association.

Steigerwald, F., & Stone, D. (1999). Cognitive restructuring and the 12-Step Program of Alcoholics Anonymous. *Journal of Substance Abuse Treatment, 16*(4), 321-327. doi: 10.1016/S0740-5472(98)00052-X.

Striegel-Moore, R. H., & Bulik, C. M. (2007). Risk factors for eating disorders. *American Psychologist, 62*(3), 181-198. doi: 10.1037/0003-066X.62.3.181.

Striegel-Moore, R. H., Rosselli, F., Perrin, N., DeBar, L., Wilson, G. T., May, A., & Kraemer, H. C. (2009). Gender difference in the prevalence of eating disorder symptoms. *International Journal of Eating Disorders, 42*, 471-474. doi.org/10.1002/eat.20625.

Vandecreek, L., Nye, C., & Herth, K. (1994). Where there's life, there's hope, and where there is hope, there is… *Journal of Religion and Health, 33*, 51-59. doi: 10.1007/BF0234499.

van Manen, M. (1977). Linking ways of knowing with ways of being practical. *Curriculum Inquiry, 6*(3), 205-228.

van Manen, M. (1990). *Researching lived experience: Human science for an action sensitive pedagogy*. London, Ontario: Althouse Press.

van Manen, M. (1997). *Researching lived experience: Human science for an action sensitive pedagogy* (2nd ed.). London, Ontario: Althouse Press.

van Manen, M. (2007). Phenomenology of practice. *Phenomenology & Practice, 1*(1), 11-30.

von Ranson, K. M., Russell-Mayhew, S., & Masson, P. C. (2011). An exploratory study of eating disorder psychopathology among Overeaters Anonymous members. *Eating & Weight Disorders, 16*, e65-e68. doi: 10.1007.BF03327524.

von Ranson, K. M., Wallace, L. M., & Stevenson, A. (2013). Psychotherapies provided for eating disorders by community clinicians: Infrequent use of evidence-based treatment. *Psychotherapy Research, 23*(3), 333-343. doi: 10.1080/10503307.2012.735377.

von Ranson, K. M., & Farstad, S. M. (2014). Self-help approaches in the treatment of eating disorders, substance use disorders, and addictions. In T. D. Brewerton & A. B. Dennis (Eds.), *Eating Disorders, addictions and substance use disorders: Research, clinical and treatment perspectives* (pp. 587-608). Heidelberg, Berlin: Springer.

Wampold, B. E. (2015). How important are the common factors in psychotherapy? An update. *World Psychiatry, 14*(3), 270-277. doi: 10.1002/wps.20238.

Wasson, D. H. (2003). A qualitative investigation of the relapse experiences of women with bulimia nervosa. *Eating Disorders, 11*(2), 73-88. doi: 10.1080/10640260390199271.

Wasson, D. H., & Jackson, M. (2004). An analysis of the role of Overeaters Anonymous in women's recovery from bulimia nervosa.

Eating Disorders, 12(4), 337-356. doi: 10.1080/10644026049052 1442.

Wetzler, S., Hackmann, C., Peryer, G., Clayman, K., Friedman, D., Saffran, K., Silver, J., Swarbrick, M., Magill, D., van Furth, E. F., & Pike, K. M. (2020). A framework to conceptualize personal recovery from eating disorders: A systematic review and meta-synthesis of perspectives from individuals with lived experience. *International Journal of Eating Disorders, 53*(8), 1188-1203. doi: 10.1002/ eat.23260.

Williamson, D. A., Martin, C. K., & Stewart, T. (2004). Psychological aspects of eating disorders. *Best Practice & Research Clinical Gastroenterology*, *18*(6), 1073-1088. doi: 10.1016/j.bpg.2004.06.023.

Wonderlich, S., Mitchell, J. E., Crosby, R. D., Myers, T. C., Kadlec, K., LaHaise, K., Swan-Kremeier, L., Dokken, J., Lange, M., Dinkel, J., Jorgensen, M., & Schander, L. (2012). Minimizing and treating chronicity in the eating disorders: A clinical overview. *International Journal of Eating Disorders, 45*(2), 467-475. doi: 10.1002/eat.20978.

Wright, k. M., & Hacking, S. (2012). An angel on my shoulder: A study of relationships between women with anorexia nervosa and healthcare professionals. *Journal of Psychiatric and Mental Health Nursing, 19*, 107-115. doi: 10.1111/j.1365-2850.2011.01760.x.

Yalom, I. D. (2005). *The theory and practice of group psychotherapy* (5th ed.). New York: Basic Books.

Yeary, J. (1987). The use of Overeater's Anonymous in the treatment of eating disorders. *Journal of Psychoactive Drugs, 19*(3), 303-309. doi: 10.1080/02791072.1987.10472417.

In: A Closer Look at Women's Health ISBN: 978-1-68507-408-1
Editor: Lakisha Roberts

Chapter 2

The Effects of Hope and Body Shame on Alcohol and Drug Use in Eating Disordered Women

Jennifer A. Boisvert[1,*] and W. Andrew Harrell[2]
[1]Independent Practice, Beverly Hills, CA, USA
[2]University of Alberta, Edmonton, Alberta, Canada

Abstract

The eating disorder literature has not adequately considered the importance of hope as a mediating factor in the complicated relationships between body shame and eating disorder behavior, nor its relationship with substance use/abuse behavior. To provide more clarity, an Internet survey of women (N = 297) examined substance use/abuse (alcohol and drugs) as a function of body shame, hope, and eating disorder symptomatology. Twenty-percent reported treatment for an eating disorder at some time; 10% had been treated for anorexia nervosa (AN), with 8.1% treated for bulimia nervosa (BN). Forty-six percent had been treated for both AN and BN.

* Corresponding Author's E-mail: jenniferboisvert@hotmail.com.

Most had been treated within the last two years (49%), but fully 22% had been treated 6 years or more in the past. Seventy-seven percent of the sample reported alcohol use/abuse, and 76% non-medical drug use/abuse. Structural equation modeling (Lavaan, SEM) tested a series of models, finding that hope and body shame were critical mediators, linking eating disorder symptomatology (EAT-26) to women's alcohol and drug use/abuse behavior. Hope was the dominant factor. Women treated for AN were more impacted by variations in hope. BNs had either direct links to substance use/abuse, or had an effect mediated by eating disorder symptomatology. The implications of these findings for research and practice are discussed.

Keywords: women, eating disorders, hope, body shame, substance use, alcohol use, drug use

INTRODUCTION

Hope is an important concept for understanding the development and maintenance of eating disorder symptomatology, i.e., eating disorder attitudes and behaviors. In the previous chapter, Boisvert (2021) shows that the experience of hope in a 12-Step self-help group can be critical for women's recovery from clinical eating disorders of anorexia nervosa (AN) and bulimia nervosa (BN). It shows that in real-time there is a process by which hope emerges from group interactions and fellowship in the 12-Step program that alters the thinking and feeling of AN and BN women. The fact that hope was instilled, maintained, and projected in the 12-Step group suggests that hope is in essence a social-relational construct, enhancing healthier behavior, including substances disuse among women reporting co-morbid alcohol and/or drug use. In this chapter, we expand our exploration of hope, and how it is an important mediating variable, connecting women's eating disordered behavior with their substance use/abuse behavior.

Hope

Hope is a cornerstone of physical, psychosocial, and spiritual health and well-being (Snyder, Irving, et al., 1991). Hope has relevance for the development of eating disturbances and disorders in girls and women (Irving & Cannon, 2000). Higher hope, i.e., hopefulness, has many health benefits, including adaptive coping and optimal functioning (Snyder, 1994, 1999). A hopeful person is one who actively sets and attains general or specific future goals, despite fluctuating situations, challenges, or barriers (Snyder, 2000; Snyder, Ilardi, et al., 2000).

In Snyder's (1994) hope theory, people are guided by efforts to reach and obtain goals. Hope, as defined in Snyder's (1994) model, is "the process of thinking about one's goals, along with the motivation to move toward (agency) and the ways to achieve (pathways) these goals" (Snyder, 1995, p. 355). In this model, hope is conceptualized as a "will" to attain a desired outcome, and a "way" of mobilizing resources and coping. Agency, also called "will," is a sense of purpose or determination that one has in terms of meeting short- and long-term goals. Agency directs positive mental energy along pathways when one is faced with obstacles or challenges in moving towards achieving a set goal(s). When faced with blockages to their goals, agency helps people to channel the requisite motivation to the best alternate pathway. Pathways, also called "way," are plans or strategies through which future goals can be achieved and desired outcomes attained. Pathways may occur in the form of engaged coping efforts, such as problem-solving, that better enable one to be successful in achieving a set goal(s). Hoping and coping are theorized as having a relationship wherein they build onto and into each other (Snyder, 1994, 2000).

Hope and Substance Use/Abuse

Little attention has been given to the impact of hope on substance use/abuse or more severe addictions or substance use disorders such as alcoholism and/or illicit drugs, e.g., heroin.

Irving et al. (1998) examined hope and recovery from substance dependence in homeless veterans ($N = 90$). Higher hope was related to longer abstinence and better quality of life as well as greater self-efficacy. Higher hope was also correlated with more recovery-related variables.

Mathis et al. (2009) examined relationships between hope and substance use abstinence in communal-living recovery home residents ($N = 90$). Linear regression analyses suggested that hope might be linked to substance use at later stages of recovery. Results also suggested a stronger relationship between hope and drug use than alcohol use.

Law and Guo (2012) found that a hope-based substance abuse treatment program, designed to help women drug offenders ($N = 40$), resulted in greater recovery compared to a control group ($N = 20$). Analysis of covariance (ANCOVAs) showed that hope increased more in the women drug offenders who completed the program than in the control group; significant differences in their ability to cope were also observed.

More recently, Gutierrez (2019) examined relationships between meaning in life, hope, and spiritual experiences on alcohol and drug use severity in a community sample of women and men ($N = 406$). Structural equation models (SEM) showed a significant relationship between meaning in life and alcohol and drug use severity. Hope was shown as having both a direct effect on alcohol and drug use severity, and a mediator between spiritual experiences and meaning in life.

Hope, Body Shame, and Eating Disorder Symptomatology

The research on hope and eating disorder behavior is sparse, and much of it comes from our program of research. In this chapter we explore linkages between hope, body shame, and eating disorder behavior that may impact women's substance use/abuse behavior.

Body Shame and Eating Disorder Symptomatology

Our research has described body shame as a pivotal variable, leading to eating disorder symptomatology (Boisvert, 2006; Boisvert & Harrell, 2009). Body shame has been shown to be a motivator for women's use of harmful weight control behaviors such as dieting, use of laxatives, or purging via vomiting or excessive exercise (Fredrickson & Roberts, 1997; McKinley & Hyde, 1996). Higher body shame may lead to expressions of eating disorder symptomatology in women, especially for those with higher body mass index (BMI), i.e., heavier weight (Boisvert, 2006; Boisvert & Harrell, 2009; Frederick & Grow, 1996; Fredrickson et al., 1998; Noll & Fredrickson, 1998; Slater & Tiggemann, 2002; Tiggemann & Slater, 2001).

Hope, Body Shame, and Eating Disorder Symptomatology

Hope and body shame can interact to have a complicated relationship to eating disorder symptomatology. Women who scored lower on two measures of hope tended to have higher body shame and, subsequently, greater eating disorder symptomatology. This was especially strong in women with higher (BMI) (Boisvert, 2006; Boisvert & Harrell, 2013). This relationship can be further complicated by other variables such as greater severity of eating behaviors, i.e., clinical eating disorders. Boisvert (2001) investigated the relationship between level of hope and eating disorder symptom severity in women with clinical eating disorders ($N = 31$; AN $n = 17$, BN $n = 14$) and a control group of women ($N = 31$). T-tests showed that eating disordered women had lower hope than the control group. Correlation analyses showed a relationship between lower hope and greater eating disorder symptom severity.

Eating Disorder Symptomatology and Substance Use/Abuse

Substance use/abuse, i.e., addiction, has received considerable attention its relationship to eating disorders (von Ranson & Cassin, 2007). Reviews of the co-morbidity of eating disorders and substance use disorders document that these disorders frequently co-occur, particularly in women with bulimia nervosa (BN), or binge eating/purging subtype of anorexia nervosa (AN-BN and PAN) (for reviews, see Bahji et al., 2019; Harrop & Marlatt, 2010; Nøkleby, 2012.) BN women or AN women with bulimic features, e.g., purging, are generally more likely to report alcohol and drug use/abuse than AN women with restricting behavior (RAN) (Krug et al., 2008; for review, see Gadalla & Piran, 2007). Studies of substance use prevalence find differences across AN subtypes, with AN-BN women, especially those with bulimic features who purged, reporting substance use more than AN women who only restricted or purged (Krug et al., 2009; Root et al., 2010). Lifetime substance abuse may be more prevalent in AN women with bulimic features, e.g., binge eating, as a function of higher novelty-seeking or impulsivity (Fernández-Aranda et al., 2007; Krug et al., 2009). Higher novelty-seeking might explain diagnosis cross-over (Krug et al., 2009). Lifetime impulse control disorders often presents in women with binge eating subtypes, given their tendency to report using laxatives, diuretics, appetite suppressants, and fasting—all of which have been associated with more eating psychopathology and pathological personality traits (Fernández-Aranda et al., 2007). Research examining prevalence of personality disorders and features in eating disorder subgroups suggests AN women have high constraint and persistence, and low novelty-seeking, while BN women have high impulsivity, sensation-seeking, novelty-seeking, and traits associated with borderline personality disorder (for review, see Cassin & von Ranson, 2005). That is, BN women appear to have a more impulsive, addictive personality than AN women, except those AN women with bulimic features.

Substance use/abuse behavior in women might be maintained because of its negative reinforcing features. As a whole it might reduce body-related anxiety/stress, e.g., body image disturbance, or distract them from acting on binge eating impulses/urges (Fernández-Aranda et al., 2007; Krug et al., 2009)

Substance Use/Abuse as Anxiety/Stress Reduction

Studies of individual-level motives for substance use/abuse behavior have hypothesized that it is a means of reducing stress, anxiety, or depression (Granner et al., 2002). In a nonclinical sample of college women (N = 206), Granner et al. (2002) observed that escape drinking was associated with heavier drinking. Granner et al. (2002) also noted that eating disorder symptomatology, notably body dissatisfaction and drive for thinness, were statistically associated with heavy drinking. Linear regression analyses showed escape drinking accounted for a greater increase in explained variance in body dissatisfaction and drive for thinness than for BMI. The results suggested that BMI had a lesser, indirect effect on drive for thinness, mediated by body dissatisfaction. Granner et al. (2002) opined that dissatisfaction with body shape, as well as the pursuit of thinness, were expressions of eating disorder symptomatology that generated anxiety, and that this anxiety motivated subsequent eating disorder behavior and alcohol abuse.

Other studies in nonclinical samples of college women, have also found binge drinking was related to dietary restraint, coping by using substances, and enhancing mood, suggesting that binge drinking is prevalent in women at risk for eating disorder behavior, or is a motive for use in those endorsing BN purging subtype and BED (e.g., Khalylis et al., 2009; Luce et al., 2007).

A New Model

The model tested in this chapter is presented in Figure 1. In this model, we hypothesize that eating disorders, particularly women with anorexia, will take an indirect pathway, through body shame, hope, and eating disorder symptomatology (represented by our abbreviated form of the EAT-26 scale), to arrive at varying degrees of alcohol and drug use/abuse. That is, anorexic women who have both lower hope and greater body shame will express this in the form of greater severity of eating disorder symptomatology; in turn, greater severity of alcohol and drug use is more likely in these women if eating disorder symptomatology is expressed. Conversely, anorexic women with higher hope will have lower body shame, lower severity of eating disorder symptomatology, and, subsequently, lesser alcohol and drug use severity.

Bulimic women may also have the indirect paths outlined above; however, there is evidence that this serious form of eating disorder may also directly impact alcohol and drug use, in part, bypassing the intervening links. This direct linkage should be found when bulimia nervosa is part of a general addictive personality. We hypothesize that the combined indirect and direct paths for bulimic women should exceed the combined effects for anorexic women, thereby affirming the often-reported finding that bulimic women exceed anorexic women in serious forms of alcohol and drug use/abuse.

Purpose of the Study

The purpose of this study was to test the hypothesized model in Figure 1 using structural equation modeling (SEM). This study differed from previous research by: (1) testing an original SEM model of eating disorders, (2) examining pathways between hope, body shame, and eating disorders, (3) examining hope and body shame in relation to alcohol and drug use/abuse.

METHOD

Internet Survey

An Internet survey on eating disorders and substance use/abuse behavior was designed (containing 49 questions total). It was then circulated on the Internet using multiple outlets and sources. These included: social media (e.g., Twitter), websites (e.g., public relations news blasts on research surveys, eating disorder organization's research web pages, the first author's research web page), and e-mail mail-outs (e.g., eating disorder organization's electronic newsletters). The survey was constructed through the LimeSurvey software, and was available worldwide to any adult over the age of 18 years. Prior to its distribution, the survey was reviewed and approved by the University of Alberta's Institutional Review Board (IRB). Although their responses remained anonymous, respondents were asked to give informed consent prior to their participation in the survey; respondents attested to being 18 years or older and gave consent by clicking a "consent button" that accessed the survey on another web page, permitting them to proceed with responding.

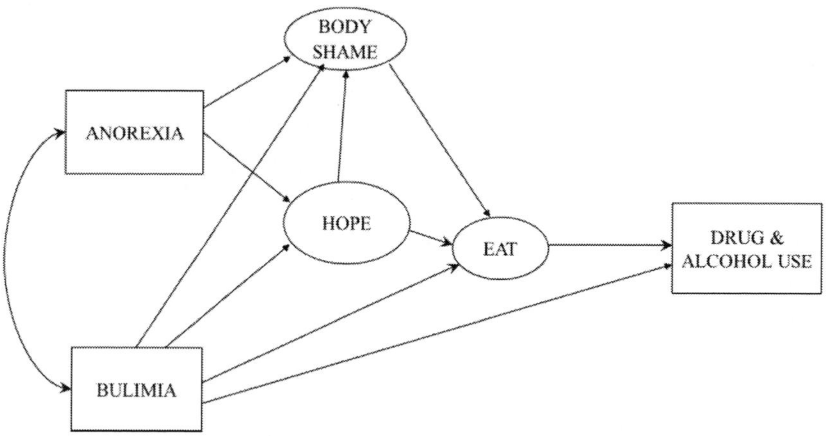

Figure 1. Proposed SEM model for anorexia-bulimia impact on alcohol and drug use.

The survey gathered general demographic information concerning respondent's age, gender, sexual orientation, level of education, marital status, race/ethnicity, and place of birth (geographic region), and current residency. Data were also obtained concerning a respondent's height and weight, "ideal" weight, and perception of her current weight status.

The variables of interest in the present study composed the bulk of the survey and dealt with body shame, hope, and eating disorders and related symptomatology, as well eating disorder treatment that may have been received, type of eating disorder treated, and a series of items dealing with substance use/abuse in the form of alcohol use, drug use, and tobacco use. Only the data on alcohol use and drug use have been analyzed in the present study. Ending the survey instrument were questions on treatment for history of depression and open-ended questions on the topic of eating disorders. These data have not been examined in this chapter.

Sample

The respondents analyzed in this chapter are not representative of any particular population. Participation was self-initiated, in response to announcements concerning the survey posted on websites or social media, as well as on other platforms open to the public on the Internet. The intent of our analysis was not to make inferences concerning eating disorders or alcohol or drug use/abuse or addictive behavior to a general clinical or nonclinical population, but, rather, to test the hypotheses outlined above in the Introduction section of this chapter.

A total of 374 respondents completed all or part of our survey. Two hundred and ninety-seven of the respondents were women, and 52 were men. Twenty-five respondents failed to identify their gender, and have been excluded. Only data provided by the women as a subgroup have been analyzed for the purpose of this study. Another reason for deferring the analyses of the men in our survey is that their numbers were smaller, creating serious difficulties for statistical analyses.

Measures

Demographic Variables

Data on the respondent's gender, date of birth, place of birth, current residency, self-identified race/ethnicity, sexual orientation, marital status, highest level of education, height and weight, ideal weight, diagnosis and treatment for an eating disorder and/or depression, and an open-ended question on personal experiences with body image, eating disorders, and substance use behaviors involving alcohol, drugs, and tobacco.

Eating Disorder Variables

Respondents were asked an initial question of whether or not they had ever been treated for an eating disorder. In follow up questions, they were asked if they had ever been treated specifically for anorexia nervosa (AN), bulimia nervosa (BN), binge eating disorder (BED), or obesity. For analysis, three dummy variables were created. In the first variable, contrasting respondents who had been treated for any eating disorder with those who had not, a categorical value of 1 was assigned to all of those treated for any kind of disorder, at any time. They were compared to those who had never been treated; this respondent category was assigned a value of 0. The second variable contrasted AN treated respondents, who were assigned a category value of 1, with all other respondents, who were given a category value of 0. In the third dummy variable, respondents treated for BN were given a value of 1, with a value of 0 for all others.

Eating Disorder Symptomatology

Eating disorder symptomatology was measured with one of the most widely used instruments the abbreviated version of the Eating Attitudes Test—Eat-26 (Garner et al., 1982). The EAT-26 has been demonstrated to be highly reliable and valid as diagnostic screening tool in nonclinical and clinical samples (for review, see Garfinkel & Newman, 2001). Studies examining the EAT's factor structure suggest it taps general eating pathology as well as more specific factors (e.g., Rogoza et al., 2016). Factor analyses have yielded a dominant factor I which primarily applies to sufferers of anorexia, as distinguished from bulimics. This factor taps into the inherent body dissatisfaction of those with anorexia nervosa, which distinguishes them from other eating disorders (Garner et al., 1982). The EAT-26 as an index of subclinical anorexia nervosa has also been validated on nonclinical samples (Button & Whitehouse, 1981). Each of the items in the EAT-26 has six response categories ranging from

Always (1) to Never (6). Because of the attenuation of cases in our survey because of numerous non-responses, for purposes of analysis in this chapter, the EAT-26 items were factor analyzed, and the items with factor loadings of at least 0.60 on the dominate factor I were identified and singled out. These selected items were incorporated into a 12-item scale in which each item was weighted by its non-rotated factor loading, and then added. This is a recommended practice for obtaining indices in which more important indicators of an underlying concept are given more value than indicators that have a weaker relationship to the property being measured, in this case, eating disorder symptomatology (DiStefano et al., 2009). The authors of the EAT-26 have indicated that a scale based on factor I weightings can be substituted for the EAT-26 (Garner et al., 1982, p. 877).

Body Shame

Body shame was measured using the Body Shame subscale of the Objectified Body Consciousness scale (OBC: McKinley & Hyde, 1996). The BS subscale consists of 8 items related to feelings of shame associated with the failure of one's body to conform to an ideal (McKinley & Hyde, 1996). Items are rated on a Likert-style scale with response categories ranging from a value of one (strongly disagree) to seven (strongly agree). A higher score reflects greater body shame. The BS subscale demonstrated adequate internal consistency for the present study sample. In order to carry out correlational analysis and tests of significance, a body shame index was created by first factor analyzing the survey participants' responses and taking the subsequent non-rotated factor loadings to weight the value of the item, and then adding them together for the index. The factor analysis revealed one major factor, accounting for 42.56% of the variance. A minor second factor accounted for 11.74%.

Hope

Hope was measured using the Hope Scale (HS: Snyder, Harris et al., 1991). The HS is a 12-item measure of hope that reflects cognitive-behavioral dimensions. As such it has two subscales: Agency (one's perceptual ability to initiate and sustain movement along chosen pathways) and Pathways (one's ability to generate avenues for attaining goals). HS items are rated across a 4-point Likert-type index ranging from a value of one (definitely false) to four (definitely true). (Two filler HS items were not included.) A higher HS total score reflects greater hopefulness. Again, a factor analysis revealed a single, dominant factor accounting for 37.47% of the variance, with two minor factors. A hope index was constructed by weighting each item by its non-rotated factor loading, and then adding.

Alcohol Use

The Brief Michigan Alcohol Screen Test (bMAST) is a 10-item test derived from the larger 25-item Michigan Alcohol Screen Test, with well-established validity as a measure of alcohol use/abuse (Connor et al., 2007). Items included whether one felt they were a normal drinker, had ever attended an Alcoholics Anonymous (AA) meeting, had lost friends because of drinking, etc. Respondents were asked to answer "yes" (1) or "no" (2) for each item. For the correlational analyses, items were added to form an index.

Drug Use

The Drug Abuse Screening Test (DAST-10) was used to measure respondent's involvement with non-medical drugs, excluding alcohol and tobacco, during the past 12 months. This is a uni-dimensional scale with strong reliability and validity (Evren et al., 2013). Response categories to the 10 items were either "yes" (1) or "no" (2). As was the case with the bMAST, items were added to form an index. Items included whether the respondent had used drugs other than for medical reasons, whether more than one drug at a time were abused, whether one had neglected their family because of drug use, etc.

Analyses

Structural Equation Modeling (SEM)

Analyses of the hypotheses were performed using the Lavaan structural equation modeling (SEM) R package (see Rosseel, 2012). SEM has been used in a number of studies of eating disorder symptoms and behaviors in adolescent girls (e.g., Neumark-Sztainer, Wall, Perry, et al., 2003; Neumark-Sztainer, Wall, Story, et al., 2003), as well as in our own research program (e.g., Boisvert, 2006; Boisvert & Harrell, 2016). This analytic approach features the ability to statistically judge the goodness-of-fit of the hypothesized model to the actual data. It also provides estimates of the strength and significance of the direct "paths" between variables within the model, as well as the indirect paths. As recommended by Kline (1998), all insignificant paths were "trimmed," i.e., that is, those not statistically significant at the .05 level or better were dropped. This trimming resulted in a more parsimonious final model. In brief, our approach was to first assess the overall model presented in Figure 1, and then calculate a final, trimmed model in which only statistically significant direct paths have been retained.

RESULTS

Descriptive Statistics

A total of 297 women participated in this online survey. Because of numerous incomplete answers to some of the survey questions, the effective sample size available for analysis varies, depending on the variables being examined. The median age of the sample was 29 years ($M = 32.73$, $SD = 11.56$), with a range from 12 to 75 years. Fifty percent of the sample resided in the United States, followed by 41% in Canada. The remaining 9% of the survey participants were primarily from Australia/New Zealand and Asia. This sample of women was highly educated, with 41.6 reporting having received a Bachelor's degree, and

33.5% with a Masters/Doctorate or professional degree. Forty-eight percent (n = 138) reported being single, 40.7% married or common-law married (n = 118). Eight percent (n = 22) were separated or widowed, and 3.5% were in a same-sex relationship (n = 10).

Eating Disorders

Twenty-percent reported being treated at some point in their life for an eating disorder; on the other hand, fully 80% of the sample had not been treated for an eating disorder. Forty-nine percent (n = 24) reported being treated within the last year, 22.4% within 2-5 years, and the remainder being treated six years or longer. Ten percent (n = 30) reported that they had been treated for AN, 8.1% (n = 24) for BN, and smaller percentages for binge eating disorder (BED) (3.7%), obesity (1.3%) or other eating disorders.

Body Shame, Hope, and EAT

Means and standard deviations for each of the indices are provided in Table 1, along with correlations for these variables.

Alcohol Use and Drug Use

Seventy-seven percent of the sample (n = 188/243) reported using alcohol in the last 12 months. Seventy-six percent (n = 185/243) had used prescription or non-medical drugs. Alcohol and drug use was significantly associated ($\chi2 = 8.02$, $df = 1$, $p < 0.01$).

Bivariate Associations

Treatment for AN was strongly associated with treatment for BN ($\chi 2 = 66.89$, $df = 1$, $p < 0.001$), with 46.7% of respondents who had been treated for AN had also been treated for BN at some point in their lives.

Associations between alcohol use, drug use, and treatment for eating disorders were also examined. Treatment for any eating disorder was not significantly related to using alcohol in the last 12 months ($\chi 2 = 1.19$, $df = 1$, $p = 0.27$); however, eating disorder treatment was significantly related to using prescription or non-prescription drugs ($\chi 2 = 4.63$, $df = 1$, $p < 0.05$). Eighty-eight percent of women who had been treated for an eating disorder reported using drugs ($n = 43/49$), compared to 73.1% ($n = 141/193$) of women who had not been treated.

In the case of anorexic women, there were nonsignificant associations between alcohol use ($\chi 2 = 0.33$, $df = 1$, $p = 0.56$) and drug use ($\chi 2 = 2.09$, $df = 1$, $p = 0.15$). Such was also the case for bulimic women, with nonsignificant associations for alcohol use ($\chi 2 = 1.78$, $df = 1$, $p = 0.18$) and drugs ($\chi 2 = 1.89$, $df = 1$, $p < 0.17$).

Table 1 presents bivariate Pearson correlation coefficients between the alcohol and drug indices and body shame, hope, and the short-form of the EAT-26 that we have adapted for this study. As hypothesized, body shame and hope were negatively related; i.e., those respondents expressing a feeling of body shame tended to score lower on the hope scale. Conversely, women scoring low on body shame had higher hope scores. Women with greater body shame also scored higher on the EAT-26 scale. That is, body shame was correlated with greater eating disorder symptomatology. Higher scores on body shame, as well as the EAT-26 scale, were correlated with greater drug use. Alcohol use was not significantly correlated with body shame; however, as we hypothesized, it was strongly associated with the EAT-26 ($r = 0.30$, $p < .001$). Greater alcohol use was significantly associated with greater drug use ($r = 0.42$, $p < .001$).[1]

[1] In the original survey coding of responses to alcohol and drug use/abuse items, as well as items comprising the EAT-26 and body shame indices, higher scores are representative of

Tests of Significance

Comparisons of means using t-tests showed statistically significant differences consistent with our hypotheses. Thus, women who were treated for any eating disorders were significantly more likely to report alcohol use/abuse ($t = -4.08$, $df = 183$, $p < 0.001$) ($M = 16.00$, $SD = 1.74$) than women not treated for an eating disorder ($M = 16.93$, $SD = 1.04$). Women treated for anorexia ($M = 15.81$, $SD = 1.89$) were more likely to report alcohol use/abuse than women not treated for anorexia ($M = 16.84$, $SD = 1.21$)($t = -3.41$, $df = 184$, $p < 0.01$). Bulimic women ($M = 15.94$, $SD = 1.18$) had greater alcohol use/abuse than non-bulimic women ($M = 16.79$, $SD = 1.33$)($t = -2.48$, $df = 184$, $p < 0.05$).

Body shame was significantly higher ($t = -5.59$, $df = 234$, $p < 0.001$) for women treated for an eating disorder ($M = 6.66$, $SD = 5.87$) than women who were not treated ($M = 13.40$, $SD = 7.81$). Body shame was significant higher ($t = -3.78$, $df = 272$, $p < 0.001$) in anorexic ($M = 7.07$, $SD = 6.49$) than non-anorexic women ($M = 12.74$, $SD = 7.88$), and higher for bulimic ($M = 7.49$, $SD = 6.45$) than non-bulimic women ($M = 12.54$, $SD = 7.93$; $t = -2.97$, $df = 272$, $p < 0.01$).

Hope tended to be lower, on average, in women treated for an eating disorder ($M = 12.47$, $SD = 3.52$) than in those who were not treated ($M = 13.96$, $SD = 3.85$)($t = -2.43$, $df = 229$, $p < 0.05$). Such was also the case with anorexic women who had lower hope ($M = 12.15$, $SD = 3.75$) than non-anorexic women ($M = 13.85$, $SD = 3.76$)($t = -2.26$, $df = 233$, $p < 0.05$). Hope was lower for bulimic versus non-bulimic women, though not statistically significant ($M = 13.11$, $SD = 4.04$ vs. $M = 13.70$, $SD = 3.79$; $t < 1$, ns).

Eating disordered women were more likely to report drug use/abuse ($M = 17.55$, $SD = 2.78$) than women who were not treated for an eating

---

lower alcohol and drug use, as well as lower EAT-26 and body shame scores on the respective indices. Correspondingly, lower cumulative scores on the indices are representative of greater alcohol and drug use, as well as lower EAT and body shame scores. In order to improve readability and interpretation in the correlation and SEM analyses, the direction of associations reported in Table 1 and in SEM Figures have been adjusted.

disorder ($M = 19.03$, $SD = 1.92$)($t = -3.93$, $df = 179$, $p < 0.001$). A similar significant difference ($t = -4.60$, $df = 179$, $p < 0.001$) was found for drug use/abuse in anorexic ($M = 16.88$, $SD = 2.98$) than non-anorexic women ($M = 16.97$, $SD = 1.94$). This was also the case for bulimic versus non-bulimic women ($M = 17.10$, $SD = 2.95$ vs. $M = 18.89$, $SD = 2.04$; $t = -3.59$, $df = 179$, $p < 0.01$).

SEM Analyses

A series of SEM analyses were carried out. These models include both manifest and latent variables. Alcohol and drug use/abuse were endogenous variables, measured by the indices constructed from the contingent questions in the survey. Anorexia treatment and Bulimic treatment were measured, exogenous variables. Body Shame, Hope and EAT have been regarded as latent variables, indexing larger, more expansive concepts. As a result the items making up the Body Shame, Hope and EAT scales in the SEM analyses have been treated as indicia of the underlying latent variable. In evaluating each model, estimates of the respective latent variable indicators have been generated by the Lavaan software. Traditionally, these indicators are produced as data in the accompanying figures, pictorially representing the models being tested. Because of the large numbers of indicators comprising our scales, however, these estimated values have been provided in tabular form, and the reader can reference them in Tables 3-5. We believe that this departure from the usual display of structural equation model estimates provides a more readable, less cluttered picture of the interconnecting paths. The reader is invited to examine these tables to assess the relative importance of individual indicators for the underlying latent concepts.

Figure 1 represents in graphic form the hypotheses tested using the R program Lavaan SEM software package. The central focus in this chapter is on a comparison of women treated at some time in their lives for anorexia or bulimia. As we pointed out earlier, these diagnoses are not mutually exclusive, with 46.7% of our respondents reporting treatments for both. The Lavaan SEM permits us to statistically isolate the unique contributions of the respective diagnoses and treatments of anorexia versus bulimia on alcohol and drug use.

Table 1. Pearson correlations

	Body Shame	Hope	Eat	Alcohol	Drugs
Body Shame	1				
Hope	-.53***	1			
Eat	.76***	-.50***	1		
Alcohol	.14	-.19*	.30***	1	
Drugs	.29***	-.25***	.37***	.42***	1
M	12.12	13.64	39.85	16.72	18.69
SD	7.93	3.81	12.18	1.34	2.23

*$p < 0.05$, **$p < 0.01$, ***$p < 0.001$

Table 2. Goodness-of-fit test results for SEMS

Goodness-of-fit Index	Alcohol Use		Drug Use	
	ANOR-BUL	All ED	ANOR-BUL	All ED
CFI	0.83	0.83	0.83	0.84
TLI	0.82	0.82	0.82	0.83
RMSEA	0.08*	0.08*	0.08*	0.08*
SRMR	0.08*	0.08*	0.07*	0.07*

CFI = Comparative Fit Index; TLI = Tucker-Lewis Index; RMSEA = Root Mean Square Error of Approximation; SRMR = Standardized Root Mean Square Residual; ED = Eating Disorders

*Acceptable fit.

Table 3. Estimated values for latent variable SHAME in trimmed models for alcohol use and drug use

SHAME Indicator	Alcohol Use	Drug Use
B01	.81 (.82)	.80 (.80)
B02	.75 (.76)	.74 (.74)
B03	.81 (.82)	.81 (.81)
B04	.76 (.76)	.76 (.76)
B05	- .66 -(.66)	-.71 (-.70)
B06	-.47 (-.47)	-.53 (-.53)
B07	.74 (.74)	.75 (.76)
B08	.80 (.80)	.82 (.82)

* Values in parentheses are for models for all eating disorders combined. Non-parenthetical values are for models comparing AN and BN.

Table 4. Estimated values for latent variable HOPE in trimmed models for alcohol use and drug use

HOPE Indicator	Alcohol Use	Drug Use
H01	-.57 (-.57)	-.58 (-.57)
H02	-.69 (-.71)	-.69 (-.69)
H03	.49 (.49)	.49 (.49)
H04	-.69 (-.68)	-.68 (-.68)
H05	.34 (.36)	.34 (.34)
H06	-.80 (-.79)	-.76 (-.76)
H07	.09 (.10)	.18 (.18)
H08	-.76 (-.75)	-.72 (-.72)
H09	-.77 (-.77)	-.75 (-.75)
H10	-.82 (-.82)	-.78 (-.78)
H11	.42 (.42)	.43 (.43)
H12	-.73 (.-72)	-.72 (-.72)

* Values in parentheses are for models for all eating disorders combined. Non-parenthetical values are for models comparing AN and BN.

Table 5. Estimated values for latent variable EAT in trimmed models for alcohol use and drug use

EAT Indicator	Alcohol Use	Drug Use
E01	.62 (.63)	.65 (.66)
E02	.76 (.76)	.78 (.78)
E03	.76 (.77)	.76 (.76)
E10	.88 (.89)	.86 (.86)
E11	.88 (.88)	.88 (.88)
E12	.62 (.62)	.62 (.62)
E14	.82 (.84)	.82 (.82)
E17	.62 (.63)	.61 (.61)
E18	.84 (.84)	.83 (.84)
E21	.84 (.84)	.82 (.82)
E22	.71 (.71)	.70 (.71)
E23	.74 (.75)	.78 (79)
E24	.64 (.64)	.68 (.69)
E26	.59 (.62)	.65 (.65)

* Values in parentheses are for all eating disorders combined. Non-parenthetical values are for models comparing AN and BN.

To accomplish this, the naturally occurring covariance of anorexia and bulimia has been included in the models that were tested, thus statistically accounting for or controlling this overlap between AN and BN respondents.

The SEM Models

Figure 1 indicates our initial hypotheses derived from a review of the literature that women diagnosed and treated for anorexia nervosa (AN) have a different "route" to alcohol or drug use than do women with bulimia nervosa (BN). Alcohol and drug use (and abuse) in anorexic women was expected to be conditional on the mediating variables body shame, hope, and eating disorder symptomatology (EAT-26). We hypothesized that alcohol and drug use in anorexic women did not necessarily represent an overall addictive personality, but rather reflected internalized pressures/stressors related to body image issues, e.g., drive for thinness, body dissatisfaction.

Bulimic women, in contrast, were expected to have a more direct connection to alcohol and drug use, with substance abuse mirroring a general addiction problem. This does not preclude the possibility that bulimic women in our sample may also take the indirect route of body image issues, particularly since a portion of the bulimic subgroup have also been treated for anorexia.

A corollary of our first hypothesis was that the overall impact of bulimia on alcohol and drug use would be stronger than for anorexic women.

In Figure 2, the eating disorders variable has only an indirect effect on the alcohol use index (bMAST). In this first analysis, there was no support for the view that eating disorders necessarily reflect simply a greater addiction problem, with alcohol use a symptom of overall substance abuse; i.e., a direct effect of self-reported eating disorder treatment on alcohol use was not statistically significant. Instead, our mediational hypothesis that eating disorder history impacts alcohol use by working through eating disorder symptomatology (i.e., greater EAT-

26 scores) is supported. In Figure 2, women with higher EAT-26 scores were also likely to have greater body shame and lower hope.

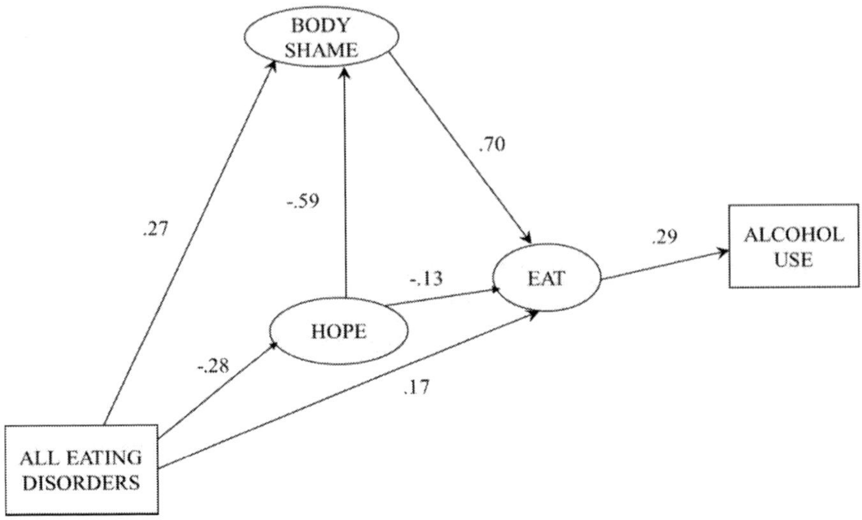

Figure 2. Trimmed SEM model for combined eating disorders and alcohol use.

Figure 3 features a test of the relationship between eating disorder treatment of any kind of eating disorder and drug use (DAST-10). Once again, a significant direct impact of eating disorders is absent, and the mediational route through body shame, hope, and EAT is again prominent. Only EAT had a direct impact on drug use. Body shame had its strongest impact on EAT; it, in turn, mediated hope and eating disorder treatment. This supports our hypothesis that hopefulness may ameliorate eating disorder symptomatology as well as body shame.

A comparison of anorexic and bulimic respondents with respect to alcohol use is shown in Figure 4. The large covariance between anorexia and bulimic subgroups represents the fact that a number of the survey participants had, at different points in their lives, been treated for both variants of eating disorder. Bulimic women in this analysis have a single path to alcohol use, though mediated by EAT. Bulimic women tended to score higher on the EAT-26, and, as a result, engaged in more alcohol use/abuse. The absence of any statistically significant direct link between bulimia and bMAST shows a lack of support for the view that bulimia is merely another form of addiction, with minor consideration given to the role that body shame, hope, and eating symptomatology might play. Anorexic women, as we hypothesized, have a more nuanced set of indirect paths, with greater body shame the contributor to a higher EAT-26 score and more subsequent alcohol use. Lower hope in anorexic women was a contributor to greater body shame. Anorexic women's use of alcohol is clearly conditional on their sense of body shame, lower hope, i.e., hopelessness, and consequent greater EAT (eating disorder symptomatology). In contrast, neither hope nor body shame was a factor in alcohol use for bulimic women.

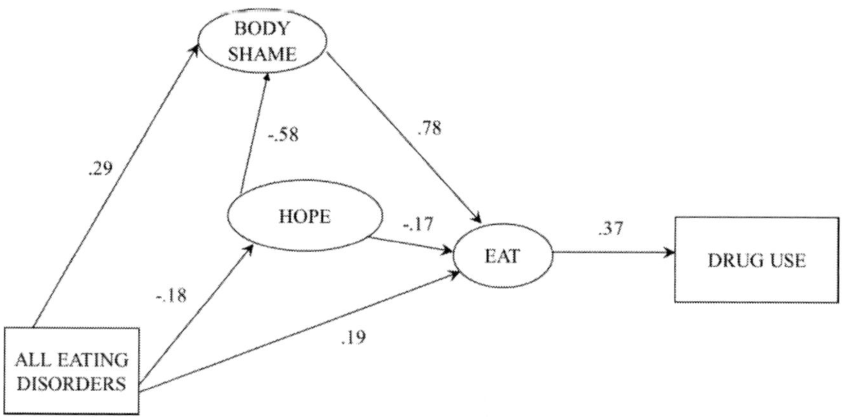

Figure 3. Trimmed SEM model for combined eating disorders impact on drug use.

Figure 5 basically repeats the findings in Figure 4—with a significant difference. Our examination of drug use finds that treatment for bulimia was a significant, direct factor in drug use, lending some support to the view that substance abuse in bulimic women might be reflective of an overall addictive personality.

Calculating Indirect Effects

To further investigate a comparison between anorexic and bulimic subgroups, total direct and indirect effects on alcohol and drug use/abuse were calculated. Calculations of these effects were guided by Barron and

Kenny (1986). In Figure 4, total indirect effects for anorexics were 0.07, based on the sum of the products of the paths for this subgroup from body shame, hope, and EAT to our indices of alcohol and drug use. In Figure 4, bulimics had a total indirect effect of 0.04; i.e., a value less than what was recorded for anorexics. This runs counter to our hypothesis (and the frequently reported observation in the literature) that BN women are more inclined to use/abuse alcohol than anorexic women because of their addictive personality features.

With Figure 5, our analysis of drug use, a much different story emerges. Anorexics only had a cumulative indirect effect of 0.03. Bulimics had an indirect effect of 0.07, but a direct effect of 0.15, for a total impact of 0.22—more than seven times the impact for anorexics. It appears then that drug use (and abuse) is more revealing of substance abuse issues for bulimics than is alcohol use/abuse.

Goodness-of-Fit Tests

Table 2 presents a number of goodness-of-fit indices for the SEM analyses. The applicability of these tests have been discussed (e.g., Chen et al., 2008; Jöreskog & Söerbom, 1988). With respect to RMSEA and SRMR, values of 0.06-0.08 are considered an acceptable fit, while values of 0.05 or less are deemed a good fit (Browne & Cudeck, 1993). Our RMSEA/SRMR values are at the upper limit of "adequate," with values of 0.07 and 0.08. These should be treated as arbitrary cutoffs or guidelines, and should not be applied without appreciating their limitations. All of the goodness-of-fit measures are strongly impacted by sample size. In the present analysis, the effective sample size was 169, and that is significantly smaller than most studies employing SEM.

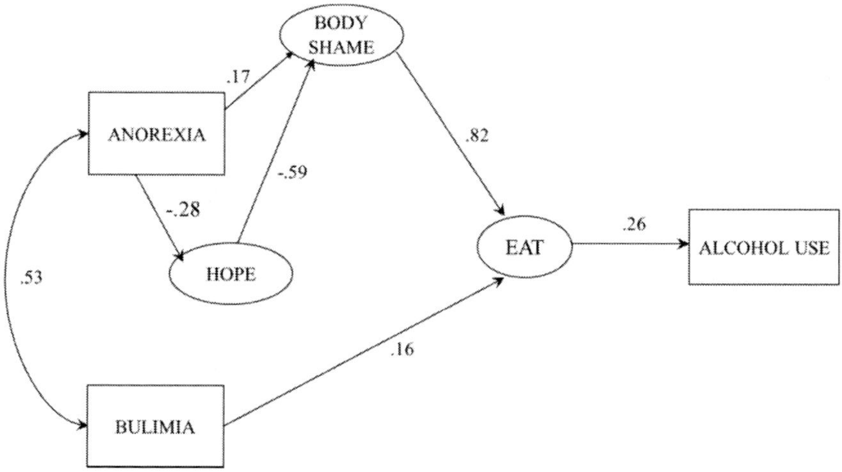

Figure 4. Trimmed SEM model for anorexia-bulimia impact on alcohol use.

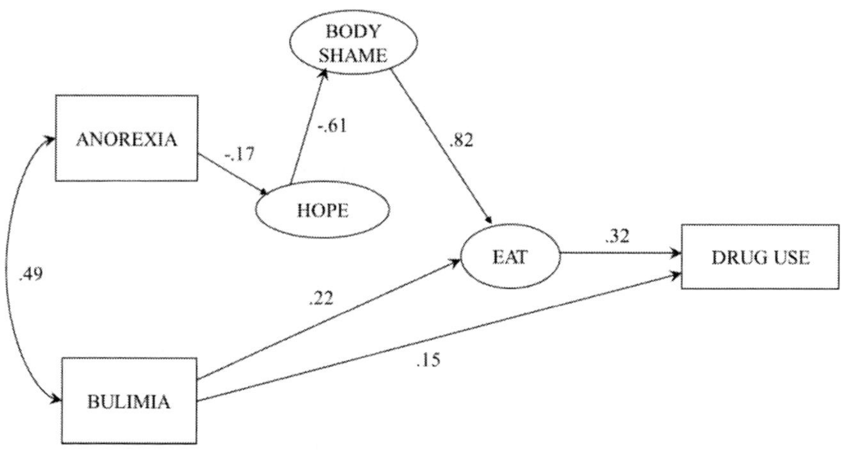

Figure 5. Trimmed SEM model for anorexia-bulimia impact on drug use.

DISCUSSION

This study makes a unique contribution to the literature, identifying novel linkages between body shame, hope, and alcohol and drug use/abuse in eating disordered women. To our knowledge, this is the first study to explore the mediational effects of hope and body shame.

Anorexics have a Different Relationship to Hope and Body Shame than Bulimics

In our SEM analysis, only those individuals who had been treated for anorexia had a significant link to the hope scale and our measure of body shame. Bulimics did not have a significant link to hope in any of the SEM analyses, nor did they have any link to body shame. Even though our original model (Figure 1) hypothesized that both anorexics and bulimics would have a significant connection to hope and body shame, in the SEM tests of the model, the links for bulimics proved to be nonsignificant. For the t-test comparisons of means, anorexics also showed a significant difference in subsample means on the hope scale between themselves and respondents who had not been treated for this eating disorder. Bulimics did not show a similar significant difference on the hope scale for either alcohol use/abuse or drug use/abuse; they did, however, show a statistically significant difference on body shame between themselves and respondents who had not been treated for an eating disorder. This difference, however, was not sustained in the SEM analyses.

In reflecting on these results, anorexics in general display a more extensive pattern of interconnected mediating variables, i.e., body shame, hope, and eating disorder symptomatology (EAT). All of the bivariate and SEM statistical analyses found that anorexics had more of a connection between their treatment status and hope and body shame, compared to respondents who reported a history of treatment for bulimia. Bulimics, in the analyses of both alcohol and drug use/abuse, showed only the single indirect connection through EAT. Bulimics, alone, had a direct impact on drug use, but not alcohol use. While this could be an artifact of the composition of our sample, we are inclined to believe that results provide a significant insight into the differing roles than hope and body shame play for patients diagnosed with AN versus BN. There are diagnostic characteristics differentiating between these eating disorders. AN is characterized by an extreme fear of weight gain and restrictive eating, while BN is characterized by bingeing then compensating for having binge eaten through purging, excessive exercise, or fasting behaviors (*DSM-5*: APA, 2013). However, these behaviors are not clear-cut, resulting in overlap or diagnostic "cross-over" or "flux," which makes it difficult to clarify or specify their relationship to study variables (Milos et al., 2005). In our analysis of anorexics, body shame captures this fear and concern over weight gain to a greater extent than for bulimics. Expressions of hopelessness by anorexics may signal an accumulating despair that fuels the sense of shame; in contrast, hopelessness may be less determinative or salient for bulimics.

Hope May Be More Important than Body Shame

It is also important to appreciate that there may be a causal ordering or sequence of hope and body shame. SEM cannot, however, determine causality in relationships. To a degree, causal ordering of the latent variables may be inferred in some cases from the relative strength of the variables. Referring to our results, in the case of alcohol use, anorexics had a stronger direct link to hope than they had to body shame. For drug use, this was also the case; indeed, the only statistically significant link (Figure 5) was between anorexic treatment status and hope. The hypothesized link between anorexic treatment status and body shame in the model for drug use/abuse was deleted in the final, trimmed model because of statistical nonsignificance.

For anorexics, what happens in terms of hopefulness is determined by their degree of body shame. In contrast, a direct link between anorexic status and body shame is weaker or lacking in statistical significance altogether. In these data, hope is the dominant variable, influencing body shame, with eating disorder symptomatology (EAT) following as a result of the hope—body shame interaction. This leads us to believe that, if participation in a self-help group or individual therapy can resolve lack of hope issues, i.e., hopelessness, body shame will likely lessen. As a consequence, eating disorder symptomatology will decline, as will substance use/abuse. This lends credence to the 12-Step approach

Boisvert (2021) describes, with its focus primarily on rehabilitating hopefulness. Body shame issues may resolve themselves along the way, but appear to have a lesser role in recovery. The final word on this can come only from closely monitored longitudinal study designs, which detect changes in hope, body shame, and eating disorder symptomatology over time. These designs could provide some verification of a true causal relationship between these variables. As it now stands, research studies are exclusively cross-sectional in nature, limiting our understanding of causal mechanisms and dynamic systems/process of eating disorders over time.

Foreshadowing the Hope—Body Shame Linkage

In 2013, we reported findings from a much larger survey-based study of eating disorder symtomatology, hope, and body shame in women (Boisvert & Harrell, 2013). We found at that time that hope also played a dominant role, mediating the impact of BMI and body shame on eating disorder symptomatology. An important finding was that hope, in some women, served as a barrier or insulator from a higher BMI manifesting as eating disorder symptomatology. Even then, we questioned that this function may differ for anorexic and bulimic women. The current chapter affirms that. The results in this chapter also extend the barrier/insulator function that we noted in 2013 to include protecting the anorexic patient from potentially harmful substance use/abuse.

The Hope—Body Shame Linkage is Significantly Different for Anorexics

Our findings shed light on how the interaction of hope and body shame might be diagnostically relevant for anorexia compared to bulimia. Boisvert's (2021) qualitative study design lacked the resources for identifying or tracking the comparative treatment or recovery success of women diagnosed with anorexic nervosa (AN), bulimia nervosa (BN) or a subtype thereof (AN-BN) of eating disorders. The results presented in this current chapter suggest that for AN women, the manifestation of eating disorder symptomatology and substance use/abuse is contingent on the interaction of hope and body shame. It appears that this is not true for BN women, however. For these women, eating disorders and substance use/abuse do not have the contingent relationship to body shame and hope. Literally, the interaction of body shame and hope is statistically irrelevant to the progression of eating disorder symptomatology and substance use/abuse in bulimics. Thus, a self-help group or individual therapy that focuses on instilling hopefulness and/or easing body shame may be more productive for AN than for other types of eating disorders, e.g., BN, BED.

The Full Spectrum of Eating Disorders Needs Study

One of the shortcomings of this study is that we were limited to comparing and contrasting anorexics and bulimics. There were just too few respondents reporting subtype combinations of anorexia and bulimia, binge eating disorder (BED), or obesity. We likely could gain a greater understanding of the hope—body shame linkage by looking at the full spectrum of eating disorders. Clearly, this limits the scope of application of our findings. In evaluating innovative treatment approaches or programs as described by Boisvert (2021), it important to assess the efficacy of hope-based treatment for different types of eating disorders.

The Full Spectrum of Substance Use/Abuse Needs Study

Again, our Internet survey method of data collection precluded asking respondents about the complete range of substance use/abuse. For example, a variety of appetite suppressors may characterize drug usage by individuals with anorexia, e.g., smoking tobacco. Bulimics may gravitate towards laxatives or substances that assist purging. Eating disordered individuals may engage in extreme behaviors related to excessive exercise and/or food/caloric intake restrictions that might be augmented by the use of certain substances. Future research that expands the range of substance use/abuse, particularly in the context of hope-focused therapy for eating disorders, may have significant therapeutic value.

Bulimia was Not More Significantly Related to Substance Use/Abuse than Anorexia

A recurrent finding in the heavily populated addiction-focused literature is that women with eating disorders engage in more substance abuse than non-eating disordered women, and that BN women have more substance-related problems than AN women. Our study did not confirm that BN women would necessarily have more substance use or abuse than AN women. Again, this may be an artifact of our self-selected Internet sample, or a limitation of our choice of indicia of alcohol and drug use/abuse, i.e., these variables were each measured by brief screening tools.

Lifelong Hopelessness?

The mean age of women in this survey was 33 years. A significant number of women had been treated for various eating disorders more than six years ago, and many were being treated in their 30s or older. Eating disorders is not just an illness for adolescent girls and young adult women, which women necessarily grow out of. Eating disorders can be chronic and of long duration. Lack of hope or hopelessness can also be long-term, even lifelong, and we believe that it is possible that in certain eating disordered women, e.g., AN restricting (RAN), AN bingeing (AN-BN), and AN purging (PAN), substance use/abuse may be means of escaping or avoiding negative emotions. If these maladaptive coping efforts prove fruitless or are experienced as repeat failures over time, AN women in particular, driven by hopelessness, may escalate their efforts in the form of suicidal gestures/attempts. In Boisvert's (2021) study, AN and BN women, too, were an average age of 37 years, had a lengthy duration of illness and series of treatments, and co-morbid alcohol and/or drug use. This is to say that for clinical eating disordered women, especially AN women, who have a greater desire to die and higher mortality due to more severe and lethal suicide attempts (Guillaume et al., 2011), chronic, unrelenting hopelessness might be a factor driving their desire for death.

Implications for Research and Practice

This study was somewhat exploratory given the novelty of the relationships examined in the SEM analyses. We recommend hypothesizing new models that might provide a broader and more informed picture of eating disorders in clinical samples of women. Future research aimed at testing statistical models, e.g., structural equation modeling (SEM), can confirm and extend research that has found complicated relationships between body shame, hope, and eating disorder symptomatology (Boisvert, 2006; Boisvert & Harrell, 2013, 2016). It could also offer more evidence of the importance of hope for eating disordered women and the use of hope-focused interventions in their treatment (Boisvert, 2001, 2021). We still lack knowledge of hope as an individual differences variable and as a social-relational construct that can uniquely impact women's healthy and unhealthy eating behaviors, as well as their successful treatment and recovery. This, indeed, is the take away from Boisvert's (2021) chapter. In her study, Boisvert (2021) found eating disordered women experienced the hope as social-relational, enhancing their recovery as participants seeking self-help in a 12-Step group as an alternative treatment. In her sample, participants also reported co-morbid alcohol and/or drug use behavior (Boisvert, 2021).

Practitioners should consider referring their patients to 12-Step programs as a treatment adjunct, especially for those patients who might have co-occurring alcohol and/or drug use problems.

Acknowledgments

Appreciation is extended to Wayne McVey, Jr., Ph.D., for his expertise in demography and population research, and to The Society for Edmonton Demographers (SED) for funding.

References

American Psychiatric Association. (2013). *Diagnostic and statistical manual of mental disorders: DSM-5* (5th ed.). Arlington, VA: Author.

Bajji, A., Mazhar, M. N., Hudson, C. C., Nadkarni, P., MacNeil, B. A., & Hawken, E. (2019). Prevalence of substance use disorder comorbidity among individuals with eating disorders: A systematic review and meta-analysis. *Psychiatry Research*, *273*, 58-66. doi: 10.1016/j.psychres.2019.01.007.

Barron, R. M., & Kenny, D. A. (1986). The moderator-mediator variable distinction in social psychology research: Conceptual, strategic, and statistical consideration. *Journal of Personality and Social Psychology*, *51*(6), 1173-1182.

Boisvert, J. A. (2001). *The relationship between level of hope and coping in eating disordered women*. Unpublished master's thesis. University of Regina, Regina, Saskatchewan.

Boisvert, J. A. (2006). The relationship between hope, coping, spirituality and eating disorder symptomatology in women. *Dissertation Abstracts International: Section B: The Sciences and Engineering*, *66*(9-B), 5078.

Boisvert, J. A., & Harrell, W. A. (2009). Ethnic and age differences in eating disorder symptomatology among Albertan women. *Canadian Journal of Behavioural Science*, *41* (3), 143-150. doi: 10.1037/ a0014689.

Boisvert, J. A., & Harrell, W. A. (2013). The effects of hope, body shame and body mass index on eating disorder symptomatology in women. *International Journal of Psychology Research*, *8*(3), 207-226.

Boisvert, J. A., & Harrell, W. A. (2016). Spirituality, religiosity and eating disorder symptomatology in women. In R. Cooper (Ed.), *Religiosity: Psychological perspectives, individual differences and health benefits* (pp. 103-192). Hauppauge, NY: Nova Publishers.

Browne, M. W., & Cudeck, R. (1993). Alternative ways of assessing model fit. In K. A. Bollen, & J. S. Long (Eds.), *Testing structural equation models* (pp. 136-162). Thousand Oaks, CA: Sage.

Button, E. J., & Whitehouse, A. (1981). Subclinical anorexia nervosa. *Psychological Medicine*, *11*(3), 509-516. doi: 10.1017/ S00332917 0005282X.

Cassin S. E., & von Ranson, K. M. (2005). Personality and eating disorders: A decade in review. *Clinical Psychology Review*, *25*, 895-916. doi: 10.1016/j.cpr.2005.04.012.

Chen, F., Curran, P. J., Bollen, K. A., Kirby, J., & Paxton, P. (2008). An empirical evaluation of the use of fixed cutoff points in RMSEA test statistic in structural equation models. *Sociological Methods & Research*, *36*(4), 462-494. doi: 10.1177/0049124108314720.

Connor, J. P., Grier, M., Feeney, G. F. X., & Young, R. M. (2007). The validity of the Brief Michigan Alcohol Screening Test (bMAST) as a problem drinking severity measure. *Journal of Studies on Alcohol and Drugs*, *68*(5), 771-779. doi: 10.15288/jsad.2007.68.771.

DiStefano, C., Zhu, M., & Mîndrilă, D. (2009). Understanding and using factor scores: Considerations for the applied researcher. *Practical Assessment, Research, and Evaluation*, *14*. doi: 10.7275/da8t-4g52.

Evren, C., Can, Y., Yilmaz, A., Ovali, E., Cetingok, S., Karabulut, V., & Muthlu, E. (2013). Psychometric properties of The Drug Abuse Screening Test (DAST-10) in heroin dependent adults and adolescents with drug use disorder. *Journal of Psychiatry & Neurological Sciences*, *26*(4), 351-359. doi: 10.5350/DAJPN2013260404.

Fernandéz-Aranda, F., Pinheiro, A. P., Thornton, L. M., Berrettini, W. H., Crow, S., Fichter, M. M., Halmi, K. A., Kaplan, A. S., Keel, P., Mitchell, J., Rotondo, A., Strober, M., Woodside, D. B., Kaye, W. H., & Bulik, C. M. (2007). Impulse control disorders in women with eating disorders. *Psychiatry Research*, *157*(1-3), 147-157. doi: 10.1016.j.psych.res.2007.02.011.

Frederick, C. M., & Grow, V. M. (1996). A mediational model of autonomy, self-esteem, and eating disordered attitudes and behaviors. *Psychology of Women Quarterly*, *20*(2), 217-228. doi: 10.1111/j.1471-6402.1996.tb00468.x.

Fredrickson, B. L., & Roberts, T. A. (1997). Objectification theory: Toward understanding women's lived experiences and mental health risks. *Psychology of Women Quarterly*, *21*(2), 173-206. doi: 10.1111/j.1471-6402.1997.tb00108.x.

Fredrickson, B. L., Roberts, T., Noll, S. M., Quinn, D. M., & Twenge, J. M. (1998). That swimsuit becomes you: Sex differences in self-objectification, restrained eating, and math performance. *Journal of Personality and Social Psychology*, *75*(1), 269-284. doi: 10.1037/0022-3514.75.1.269.

Gadalla, T., & Piran, N. (2007). Co-occurrence of eating disorder and alcohol use disorders in women: A meta-analysis. *Archives of Women's Mental Health*, *10*, 133-140.

Garfinkel, P. E., & Newman, A. (2001). The Eating Attitudes Test: Twenty-five years later. *Eating & Weight Disorders*, *6*, 1-21.

Garner, D., Olmsted, M., Bohr, Y., & Garfinkel, P. (1982). The Eating Attitudes Test: Psychometric features and clinical correlates. *Psychological Medicine*, *12*(4), 871-878. doi: 10.1017/S0033291700049163.

Granner, M., Black, D. R., & Abood, D. A. (2002). Levels of cigarette and alcohol use related to eating-disorder attitudes. *American Journal of Health Behavior*, *26*(1), 43-55. doi: 10.5593/AJHB.26.1.5.

Guillame, S., Jaussent, I., Oilié, E., Genty, C., Bringer, J., Courtet, P., & Schmidt, U. (2011). Characteristics of suicide attempts in anorexia and bulimia nervosa: A case-control study. *PLoS ONE*, *6*(8), e23578. doi: 10.1371/journal.pone.0023578.

Gutierrez, D. (2019). Spiritus contra spiritum: Addiction, hope, and the search for meaning. *Spirituality in Clinical Practice*, 1-11. doi: 10.1037/scp0000201

Harrop, E. N., & Marlatt, G. A. (2010). The comorbidity of substance use disorders and eating disorders in women: Prevalence, etiology, and treatment. *Addictive Behaviors*, *35*(5), 392-398. doi: 10.1016/j.addbeh.2009.12.016.

Irving, L. M., & Cannon, R. (2000). Starving for hope: Goals, agency, and pathways in the development and treatment of eating disorders. In C. R. Snyder (Ed.), *Handbook of hope: Theory, measures, and applications* (pp. 261-283). San Diego, CA: Academic.

Irving, L. M., Seider, A. L., Burling, T. A., Pagliarini, R., & Robbins-Sisco, D. (1998). Hope and recovery from substance dependence in homeless veterans. *Journal of Social & Clinical Psychology*, *17*(4), 389-406. doi: 10.1521/jscp.1998.4.389.

Irving, L. M., Snyder, C. R., & Crowson, J. J. Jr. (1998). Hope and coping with cancer by college women. *Journal of Personality*, *66*(2), 195-214. doi: 10.1111/1467-6494.00009.

Jöreskog, K. G., & Söerbom, D. (1988). *LISERL 7: A guide to the program and its application*. Chicago, IL: SPSS Inc.

Khaylis, A., Trockel, M., & Taylor, C. B. (2009). Binge drinking in women at risk for developing eating disorders. *International Journal of Eating Disorders*, *42*(5), 409-414. doi: 10.1002/eat.20644.

Kline, R. B. (1998). *Principles and practice of structural equation modeling.* New York: Guilford.

Krug, I., Pinheiro, A. P., Bulik, C., Jimenéz-Murcia, S., Granero, R., Penelo, E., Masuet, C., Agüera, Z., & Fernández-Aranda, F. (2009). Lifetime substance abuse, family history of alcohol abuse/dependence and novelty seeking in eating disorders: Comparison study of eating disorder subgroups. *Psychiatry and*

Clinical Neurosciences, *63*, 82-87. doi: 10.1111/j.1440-1819.01908.x.

Krug, I., Treasure, J., Anderluh, M., Bellodi, L., Cellini, E., di Bernardo, M., Granero, R., Karwautz, A., Nacmias, B., Penelo, E., Ricca, V., Sorbi, S., Tchanturia, K., Wagner, G., Collier, D., & Fernández-Aranda, F. (2008). Present and lifetime comorbidity of tobacco, alcohol and drug use in eating disorders: A European multicenter study. *Drug and Alcohol Dependence*, *97*(1-2), 169-179. doi: 10.1016/ j.drugalcdep.2008.04.015.

Law, F. M., & Guo, G. J. (2012). Hope and recovery from substance abuse for female drug offenders in Taiwan. *International Journal of Offender Therapy and Comparative Criminology*, *56*(8), 1-25. doi:10.1177/0306624X11426418.

Luce, K. H., Engler, P. A., & Crowther, J. H. (2007). Eating disorders and alcohol use: Group differences in consumption rates and drinking motives. *Eating Behaviors*, *8*(2), 177-184. doi: 10.1016/j.eatbeh. 2006.04.003.

Mathis, G. M., Ferrari, J. R., Groh, D. R., & Jason, L. A. (2009). Hope and substance use recovery: The impact of agency and pathways within an abstinent communal-living setting. *Journal of Groups in Addiction & Recovery*, *4*(1/2), 42-50. doi: 10.1080/1556035 0802712389.

McKinley, N. M., & Hyde, J. S. (1996). The objectified body consciousness scale: Development and validation. *Psychology of Women Quarterly*, *20*(2), 181-215. doi: 10.1111/j.1471-6402.1996. tb00467.

Milos, G., Spindler, A., Schnyder, U., & Fairburn, C. G. (2005). Instability of eating disorder diagnoses: Prospective study. *British Journal of Psychiatry*, *187*(6), 573-578. doi: 10.1192/bjp.197.6.573.

Neumark-Sztainer, D., Wall, M. M., Perry, C. L., & Story, M. (2003). Correlates of fruit and vegetable intake among adolescents: Findings from Project EAT. *Preventative Medicine*, *37*(3), 198-208. doi: 10.1016/S0091-7535(03)00114-2

Neumark-Sztainer, D., Wall, M. M., Story, M., & Perry, C. L. (2003). Correlates of unhealthy weight-control behaviors among adolescents: Implications for prevention programs. *Health Psychology*, *22*(1), 88-98. doi: 20.1037/0278-6133.22.1.88.

Nøkleby, H. (2012). Comorbid drug use disorders and eating disorders—A review of prevalence studies. *Nordic Studies on Alcohol and Drugs*, *29*(3), 303-314. doi: 10.2478/v10199-012-0024-9.

Noll, S. M., & Fredrickson, B. L. (1998). A mediational model linking self-objectification, body shame, and disordered eating. *Psychology of Women Quarterly*, *22*(4), 623-636. doi: 10.1111/j.1471-6402.1998.tb00181.x.

Rogoza, R., Brytek-Matera, A., & Garner, D. M. (2016). Analysis of the EAT-26 in a non-clinical sample. *Archives of Psychiatry and Psychotherapy*, *2*, 54-58. doi: 10.12740/APP/63647.

Root, T. L., Pinheiro, A. P., Thornton, L., Strober, M., Fernandéz-Aranda, F., Brandt, H., Crawford, S., Fichter, M. M., Halmi, K. A., Johnson, C., Kaplan, A. S., Klump, K. L., La Via, M., Mitchell, J., Woodside, D.B., Rotondo, A., Berrettini, W. H., Kaye, W. H., & Bulik, C. M. (2010). Substance use disorders in women with anorexia nervosa. *International Journal of Eating Disorders*, *43*(1), 14-21. doi: 10.1002/eat. 20670.

Rosseel, Y. (2012). Lavaan: An R package for structural equation modeling. *Journal of Statistical Software*, *48*(2), 1-36.

Slater, A., & Tiggemann, M. (2002). A test of objectification theory in adolescent girls. *Sex Roles*, *46*(9/10), 343-349.

Snyder, C. R. (1994). *The psychology of hope: You can get there from here*. New York: Free Press.

Snyder, C. R. (1995). Conceptualizing, measuring, and nurturing hope. *Journal of Counseling & Development*, *73*(3), 355-360. doi: 10.1002/j.1556-6676.1995.tb01764.x.

Snyder, C. R. (Ed.) (1999). *Coping: The psychology of what works*. New York: Oxford University Press.

Snyder, C. R. (Ed). (2000). *Handbook of hope: Theory, measures, and applications*. New York: Academic Press.

Snyder, C. R., Harris, C., Anderson, J. R., Holleran, S. A., Irving, L. M., Sigmon, S. T., Yoshinobu, L., Gibb, J., Langelle, C., & Harney, P. (1991). The will and the ways: Development and validation of an individual-differences measure of hope. *Journal of Personality and Social Psychology, 60*(4), 570-585. doi: 10.1037/0022-3514.60.4.570.

Snyder, C. R., Ilardi, S., Michael, S. T., & Cheavens, J. (2000). Hope theory: Updating a common process for psychological change. In C. R. Snyder, & R. E. Ingram (Eds.), *Handbook of psychological change* (pp. 128-153). New York: John Wiley.

Snyder, C. R., Irving, L. M., & Anderson, J. R. (1991). Hope and health. In C. R. Snyder, & D. R. Forsyth (Eds.), *Handbook of social and clinical psychology: The health perspective* (pp. 285-305). Elmsford, NY: Pergamon.

Tiggeman, M., & Slater, A. (2001). A test of objectification theory in former dancers and non-dancers. *Psychology of Women Quarterly, 25*(1), 57-64. doi: 10.1111/1471-6402.00007.

von Ranson, K. M., & Cassin, S. E. (2007). Eating disorders and addiction: Theory and evidence. In J. S. Rubin (Ed.), *Eating disorders and weight loss research* (pp. 1-37). Hauppauge, NY: Nova Publishers.

In: A Closer Look at Women's Health
Editor: Lakisha Roberts
ISBN: 978-1-68507-408-1

Chapter 3

INDIGENOUS AUSTRALIAN SPORTSWOMEN: INSPIRING THE NEXT GENERATION

Megan Stronach[1],* PhD, Hazel Maxwell[2], PhD and Michelle O'Shea[3], PhD

[1]Business School, University of Technology Sydney, Sydney, Australia
[2]School of Health Sciences, College of Health and Medicine, University of Tasmania, Sydney, Australia
[3]School of Business, Western Sydney University, Sydney, Australia

ABSTRACT

Sporting role models (SRM) can inspire and influence attitude and behavior. This chapter examines the influence of six Indigenous Australian sportswomen: cricketers Faith Thomas and Ashleigh Gardner, netballers Marcia Ella-Duncan and Jemma MiMi, and tennis players Evonne Goolagong-Cawley and Ashleigh Barty.

---

* Corresponding Author's E-mail: Megan.Stronach@uts.edu.au.

By applying and extending Marianne Meier's (2015) theoretical lens, it unearths and examines their role as SRMs for women and girls. Meier (2015) recognizes and describes nine functions of SRMs: participation, leadership, advocacy, challenging gender stereotypes, inspiration, ethics, safeguarding and prevention, media and corporates, and giving back. Correspondingly, Meier also identifies three categories on a 'continuum of interaction' between an observer and a successful SRM. Metaphorically the women start in silence; however, the evidence suggests that they gain—and sometimes regain—voice, often beyond their sport careers. Understanding Indigenous sportswomen's SRM status enables a layered and deep understanding of the unique platform provided by sport, which serves to strengthen their influence. The research recognizes a tenth function of female Indigenous SRMs—that of cultural maintenance. Findings illuminate how Indigenous Australian sportswomen are constructed in complex and sometimes contradictory ways, at times portrayed as advocates, deviants, sporting ambassadors, and political activists. Further research is needed to untangle the complexities and fluidity of female Indigenous Australian SRMs in the evolving worlds of both professional and community sport.

Keywords: sport role model, indigenous, Australia, sportswoman, aboriginal, empowerment

INTRODUCTION

A model can be conceived as something or someone who is endowed with visibility. In contrast, a sport role model (SRM) tends to be demarcated in moral terms. The SRM is said to inspire behaviour and attitude, thereby setting an example to follow. High-profile athletes are widely feted as public figures outside of sport, as happens with celebrities in other contexts (Dix, Phau, and Pougnet 2010). However, this is a contentious concept challenging a 'virtuous cycle of sport' (Grix and Carmichael 2012, p. 76) where, by virtue of a trickle-down effect, the broader population draws inspiration from athletes to take up or increase their sporting activities (Ishigami 2019). Yet, research shows that 'only 10 percent of elite athletes have been inspired by other elite athletes … to start with their current sport' and fewer might inspire young people to live as 'model' citizens (De Croock, De Bosscher, and van Bottenburg

2012). Accordingly, researchers remain unconvinced about the efficacy of a 'role model effect' in terms of sport engagement (Adair 2015).

While this discrepancy is recognized and acknowledged, this chapter explores how the situation is different for a small cohort of Australian sportswomen—Indigenous women and girls (Stronach, Maxwell, and Taylor 2015). Our prior scholarship led by Indigenous Australian women and utilizing culturally sensitive methodologies has demonstrated how, due partly to their sociocultural contexts, this group is unique and different from their non-Indigenous counterparts Thus for these women and girls the notion of, and necessity for SRMs has particular salience (Ferguson et al. 2019). This salience is amplified by Australian Government Shadow Minister for Families and Social Services, Aboriginal woman Linda Burney's assertions that achievements on the sporting field remain a major part of Indigenous identity in modern Australia:

> For all the challenges that confront Indigenous Australians, our Indigenous athletes provide strong role models for our youth, strengthening identity and Aboriginality, and a sense of place and belonging. And it is not so much about the physical athleticism itself, as it is about what those sporting achievements represent and the valuable lessons they have for our young people in fields beyond sport: discipline, persistence, unity, strength and dignity. (Burney 2019)

Against this backdrop, this chapter explores the experiences of six Indigenous Australian sportswomen through the history of Australian sport, specifically from the 1930s through to current times. By applying and extending Marianne Meier's (2015) theoretical lens, we shed light on, and analyze influences of, Indigenous Australian sportswomen as SRMs. Such an analysis requires an understanding of the sociocultural situations of these women, and so we start with a discussion of the on-going and pervasive effects of colonization.

BACKGROUND

While space constrains a fuller interrogation, colonization begins with one group or society taking over an area and sending people to live there. It continues with the group imposing their values or ways of life on another group, with the colonized groups expected to 'assimilate' or adopt the colonizer's ways of living. Accordingly, when Europeans arrived and settled in Australia from 1788 [considered and called by many as 'invasion' (Nicholson 2021)], Indigenous people's lives underwent forced change. They were systematically displaced, exposed to new diseases and experienced profound discrimination. Past racist legislation [e.g., the Australian *Aboriginal Protection Act* (1869)] caused great harms to Indigenous peoples. In one of the worst atrocities suffered by these people as a result of various government policies, many Aboriginal children were forcibly removed from their families. In some areas this continued until the 1970s. The children became known as the Stolen Generations (Krieken 1999). Agricultural practices introduced by settlers progressively led to a reduction in access to natural resources, as Indigenous people were displaced. Dispossession saw many Indigenous peoples rely on the provision of food from the Europeans; habitually to their detriment in terms of health and well-being (Krieken 1999). Indeed, this was an established system of segregation that inequitably shaped the lives of many Indigenous women and girls (Goodall 1995).

Together, Australian Indigenous (Aboriginal and Torres Strait Islander) peoples constitute approximately 649,200 people (2.8% of total population) (ABS, 2016). Today, the majority live in urban areas, with fewer than 25% living in remote or very remote communities. Significant sociocultural and health complexities persist for this group, including much higher child mortality rates, unemployment and criminality than in the wider population (de Leeuw, Greenwood, and Farrales 2021). Life spans are also significantly shorter among Australia's Indigenous peoples (Clarey 2000). Banned from many public gathering places, Indigenous Australians were not counted in the Australian Census until the 1967 constitutional referendum.

In the past, Aboriginal games were specific to geographic areas, although some were shared widely. Many were integral to daily life, and others were tied to ceremonies. However, the major societal changes caused by colonization stymied Indigenous peoples from participating in their traditional sports and games, and many all but disappeared (Stronach, Maxwell, and Taylor 2015). Reduction in activity levels over time, combined with poor nutrition associated with dispossession, became embedded in the social foundations and determinants of health (Gray, Macniven, and Thomson 2013). Indeed, Indigenous women in Australia have higher incidences of non-communicable diseases such as diabetes and cardiac ailments (Australian Institute of Health and Welfare 2015), for which low physical activity is a notable risk factor. Thus, for this cohort of women, exercise and sport are more than fun and games, but rather, are fundamental to realizing improved health (Reiner et al. 2013). Indigenous women's agency and power to shape imagined futures for themselves is of relevance as we look to the past and present sociocultural context. Undeniably, sport can contribute to health and social engagement (Stronach, Maxwell, and Pearce 2018), especially when led by Indigenous community members (Rowley et al. 2000).

In Australia, issues surrounding Indigenous women's and girls' sport and physical activity have increasingly received attention, signaling a potential for consideration of what part sport could play in their lives. This is despite an acknowledgment that there continues to be a lack of visible female Indigenous SRMs (Maxwell et al. 2017). A significant body of knowledge is being established which explores the status and nature of sport and physical activity for Indigenous populations (Stronach and O'Shea 2021). Much of this work notes how despite the potential benefits of sport participation, there are significant cultural and institutional constraints limiting participation (Mason and Koehli 2012), and Indigenous women's participation rates in sport and physical activity remain low (Stronach, Maxwell, and Taylor 2015).

Over 25 years ago, Colin Tatz, the most prolific Australian author to have focused on the nature of involvement of Indigenous athletes in the nation's physical culture, recognized the diabolical situation of Indigenous women. He claimed that:

> ...what black Australian woman has endured, no white woman—native or migrant—has ever endured or come close to enduring. The gradations of discrimination, the scales and dimensions of injustice, are enormous ... Of all such Cinderellas, black women's sport has the strongest case for encouragement, change, and a fair go. (Tatz 1995, pp. 98-100)

In summary, Indigenous women's involvement in sport and physical activity has reduced over time, seemingly due to external factors. Neo-colonial and neoliberal forms of domination and oppression continue to subjugate the lives of Indigenous peoples (Hayhurst, Giles, and Wright 2016). Undeniably, the pervasive effects of colonization continue to impede Indigenous women's agency, physical activity and well-being (Stronach, Maxwell, and Taylor 2015).

THEORETICAL CONCEPTS

In our introduction we signposted a definitional understanding whereby a role model is perceived as something or someone who is endowed with visibility, while a *sporting role model* is perceived in moral terms—as somebody who inspires behaviour and attitude, thereby setting an example to follow. Yet, the character and function of SRMs challenge any simplistic definitional approach. Words and phrases like 'worthy of imitation', 'inspirational', 'exemplary', and 'heroic' appear frequently in descriptors of SRMs. As already mentioned, professional and amateur athletes—whether they like it or not—rapidly become SRMs for others (Lines 2001). However, visibility and absence of *female* SRMs is frequently discussed in reports and scholarship aimed at developing female sport and/or women's and girls' empowerment through sport (Midgley et al. 2021). Furthermore, as societal values and norms diverge in these settings, the 'lack of culturally relevant role models' is identified as a significant obstacle to female sporting engagement (UN 2007, p. 18).

We also presented some words by Indigenous Australian politician Linda Burney, wherein she discusses a need for Indigenous SRMs. However, Burney's words also hint at an inherent hypocrisy in the standards that athletes as role models are expected to uphold. Accordingly, it is worth problematizing why sport is elevated to such a level that we expect someone that can run fast or hit a ball hard to behave in ways that other 'celebrities' are not expected to do. While on the field, athlete behaviour is governed by clear rules and regulations. In contrast, off-field, it is suggested 'some athletes are [to their detriment] effectively being required to be moral exemplars, to be the best citizens of all, in everything they do, at all times. No other profession is so accountable' (Jonson cited in Parker 2015, n.p.). Herein lies the contradiction, as the SRM role is clearly one that is sought after and embraced by Indigenous women. One explanation for this may be, as expressed by Indigenous Australian playwright, Andrea James, that Aboriginal women 'can't move through the world without the weight of the politics around us' (cited in O'Shea, Stronach, and Maxwell 2020, n.p.). Nonetheless, participants in our prior scholarship consistently discussed and emphasized the importance of female Indigenous SRMs, even demonstrating how Indigenous sportswomen and girls will search beyond the sport milieu to locate women who, they believe, can inspire their families and communities (Stronach, Maxwell, and Taylor 2015).

The commentary presented so far has shed light on the societal discourses and norms shaping the low participation rates of Indigenous Australian women in sport. Several influences may redress inequities, including the inspiration generated by SRMs. The value of high-profile SRMs to promote women's participation in sport is widely accepted as important (Meier 2015, Stronach, Maxwell, and Pearce 2018). However, we theorize how, due to their sociocultural situations referred to earlier, Indigenous women and girls have needs that are unique and different from their non-Indigenous counterparts, and thus the notion of, and necessity for SRMs has increased salience.

In a paper examining the value of female SRMs, Marianne Meier (2015) ascribes nine functions or attributes of female SRMs; these she lists as participation, leadership, advocacy, challenging gender stereotypes, inspiration, ethics, safeguarding and prevention, media and corporates, and giving back. Meier (2015) further classifies SRMs by identifying three categories on a 'continuum of interaction' between an observer and a potential SRM. This typology reaches from 'high/intensive degree of interaction' (type 1) such as parents or mentors to 'low/no degree of interaction' (type 3) such as famous athletes; while type 2 is an in-between group with moderate interaction, but which also includes recreational coaches. Subject to the context, observers can be young participants, peers, or fans (Meier 2015). This continuum is illustrated in Figure 1.

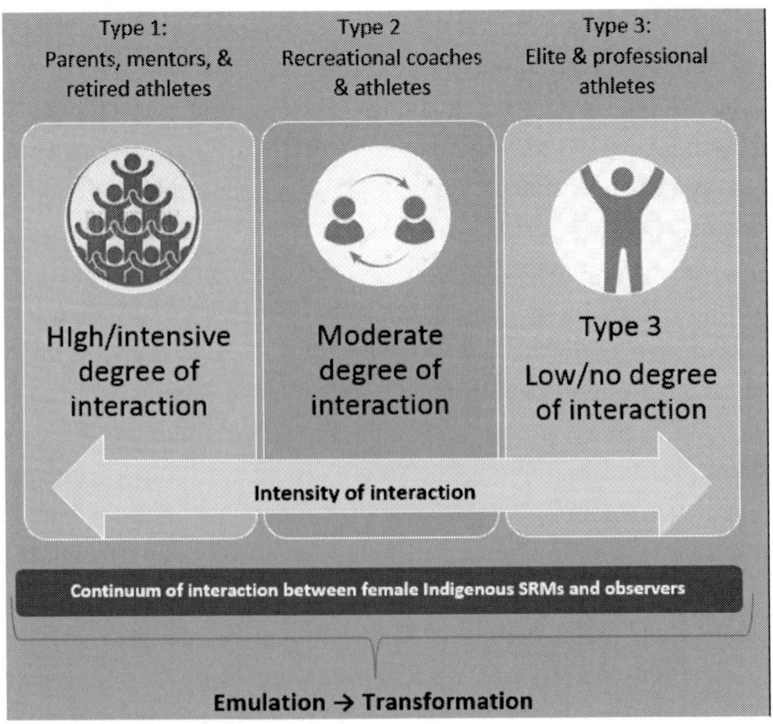

Figure 1. Continuum of interaction between female SRMs and observers.

Generally, these categories apply to any SRM, since not only high-profile athletes are effective models (Maxwell et al. 2019). Influential personalities may also come from families, local clubs, or school environments (O'Shea, Maxwell, and Stronach 2020). Some features are more likely to be evident in top-level sportswomen whereas others are manifested by recreational and higher-level coaches. The functions, attributes and features of SRMs may intersect and influence one another. Drawing from these theoretical conceptualisations, we explore the following questions:

1. What are the perceived roles and functions of female Indigenous SRMs?
2. How do Meier's (2015) theoretical models help to provide an understanding of the contested, emerging, and
3. changeable nature of these sportswomen as SRMs?

The authors of this chapter identify as non-Indigenous women. In writing about Indigenous women, we have assumed roles as active participants in cultural experiences and immersion programs both inside and outside of our university environments, and have close connections to Indigenous Australians as colleagues, research partners and friends. Through these activities we position ourselves as reflexive listeners and learners, drawing richer understandings in partnership with Indigenous colleagues.

Conceptualizing Functions of Indigenous Australian SRMs

Utilising Meier's (2015) theoretical concepts of the functions of female SRMs, the chapter outlines of the careers of six Indigenous Australian sportswomen. We consider how the women's SRM status have been constructed, navigated, and contested in complex and paradoxical ways, and often between cultures. The aim is to explore

Meier's (2015) theoretical conceptualizations of the nine functions of SRMs as well as the continuum of interaction and its application to this cohort. While by no means an exhaustive list of Indigenous Australian sportswomen, those who have been selected here form a basis for analysis. Most of the data presented derive from examination of publicly available documents, such as newspapers and magazines, images, autobiographies, literary texts, journal articles, websites, and social media.

The sportswomen who feature in our discussion are cricketers Faith (Coulthard) Thomas and Ashleigh Gardner, netballers Marcia Ella-Duncan and Jemma MiMi, and tennis players Evonne Goolagong-Cawley and Ashleigh Barty. These women's careers span from the 1930s though to current times. Some competed and are still competing at the highest echelons of professional sport, while others were active at more modest levels. The range of performance levels and behaviors both during and post-sport provide us with a rich context in which to explore narratives about Indigenous Australian sportswomen.

FAITH (COULTHARD) THOMAS

In 1958, South Australian Faith (Coulthard) Thomas became the first (and until 2019, the only) Aboriginal woman to represent Australia in cricket. In fact she was the first Indigenous Australian woman to represent Australia in any international sport (Monga 2019). Yet Thomas's greatest achievement in life was not sport related but instead came after completing her studies in midwifery and general nursing. She was among the first five Aboriginal nurses in South Australia and the state's first Aboriginal public servant (Green 2019). Before her Test cricket selection an article in her local newspaper amplifies her nursing over her sport accomplishments. Faith Coulthard was fondly described thus:

> A credit to Colebrook is Sister Faith Coulthard, who has not only succeeded in her chosen career of nursing, but has also made good on the cricket ground, being under consideration for the all-Australian team. This popular lass will be remembered by many Edenites. (Eden News, cited in Mallett 2018, p. 136)

Thomas experienced a relatively short career in elite level sport and was largely unnoticed at the time. However, sport remained central to her life; 'sport was always part of the healing process with me … and it worked' (Thomas cited in Jackson 2016). Due to cricket's amateur status (at the time) and the 'invisibility' of the women's team Thomas achieved neither great glory nor wealth. However, she certainly understood the politics of race and difference. She refused an exemption certificate, without which she was denied privileges (such as access to White sports clubs) *because* she was Aboriginal, and she remembers racist abuse (Hargreaves 2000).

Many years later, and still a feisty woman, Thomas had no qualms in calling out Australian cricketing icons Sir Donald Bradman and Lindsay Hassett for (in her eyes) not letting women's cricket prosper:

> They [men who didn't like women's cricket] were just scared of women …You look at cricket today. Australia [men's team] don't have any batsman [during the Steven Smith ban]. But women, they are just belting it all over the place. (Thomas, cited in Monga 2019)

Since her athletic retirement Faith Thomas has continually striven to give back to community, both in health care and in sport (Green 2019). Thomas became an active member of the Aboriginal Sports Foundation which she co-founded in order to 'help the up and coming sports kids who had nothing' (Tatz 1995, p. 273). Even today she is still a strong promoter of Aboriginal sport, and as an SRM she advocates for sporting opportunities for young Indigenous athletes, and continues to challenge gender norms in professional cricket (Tatz 1995). Thomas has been instrumental in the fight for Aboriginal rights and was on the management committee of the Aboriginal Legal Service in Port Augusta..

Thomas has been called 'the most important figure in Aboriginal sport' (Monga 2019). She is a culturally relevant figure who appears to embody the elements that her society holds most dear. In 2019, She was appointed a Member of the Order of Australia in the Queen's Birthday Honours List, being was recognized for significant service to cricket and to the Indigenous community Faith Thomas hopes through this award she will continue to inspire female athletes and other Indigenous leaders in the community to continue breaking boundaries (Green 2019).

ASHLEIGH GARDNER

Contemporary cricketer and world champion, Ashleigh Gardner is only the second female Indigenous cricket player to represent Australia on the international stage. She is a Muruwari woman, proud of her Indigenous background and proud that she has been able to follow in the footsteps of Faith Thomas. Ashleigh has shown qualities such as insight, leadership and activism during her cricket career and is keen to use her position as an SRM to challenge racism and empower her community by contributing to improvements in health and education. She describes her sporting career as a great privilege, 'not only do I get to represent my culture but also my country and I don't think many people get to do that especially not in cricket, I think it's just a really special thing' (Gardner, 2017).

Ashleigh is very keen to educate herself further in Indigenous culture and pass on her understanding to others—both Indigenous and non-Indigenous, for example, by leading a cultural trip of team mates to Darwin in the Northern Territory to learn more about Indigenous cultures and to participate in cultural exchange activities, in the hope of tackling cultural misunderstandings, ignorance, and racism.

> Sport is so powerful and it's been pretty cool to see what sport's been able to achieve over the last few months, with NBA teams supporting the *Black Lives Matter* movement, to the AFL signing on to

> the *Free the Flag* movement and all their teams taking a knee in their first games back after the COVID-19 shutdown. (Gardner cited in Walsh 2020)

Furthermore, she explains:

> I've been in a lot of discussions with our leadership group … giving them an insight into some of the challenges and issues facing our First Nations people and it's been really cool to be able to be involved in that, because I've never had an opportunity to talk about these things with this group before … So we'll be wearing special logos that represent Aboriginal culture on our playing shirts on Saturday, before taking off our shoes so that we're grounded to the lands, during the acknowledgement of country. (Gardner cited in Walsh 2020)

Ashleigh has created her own Foundation which links sport, health, going to school and achieving a good education. She has used her profile as a successful Aboriginal sportswoman to develop an initiative focused on providing nutritious meals, sports uniforms, and physical activity and play opportunities to young Aboriginal children. In addition to her determination to challenge barriers that young Aboriginal child might face, Ashleigh endeavors to 'give confidence and energize the next generation of little champions' (Ashleigh Gardner Foundation 2021).

Ashleigh Gardner's promotion of female Indigenous athletes is clear as she leverages her own position as an elite Indigenous sportswoman with her team, community, and her sponsors. She describes her work with these sponsors advocating for the National Indigenous Championships as 'an awesome pathway for young Indigenous cricketers' (Gardner, 2021). In support of Ashleigh's advocacy role her mother indicates that 'Ashleigh has always been really proud of being Aboriginal and as she moved up to the elite level, she knows she is a role model to others' (Gardner 2021). Her cricket teammate Alyssa Healey, supports this, portraying her colleague and friend, as 'inspiring for everyone in Australia, Indigenous or not' (Healy, cited in YouTube 2021).

MARCIA ELLA-DUNCAN

Marcia Ella-Duncan is a descendant of the Walbunja people of the far south coast of New South Wales and has kinship connections with the Bidgigal people of Botany Bay. Born in 1963, she is from the proud and famous sporting Ella family. Brothers, Glenn, Mark and Gary Ella played rugby for Australia, and Marcia was the first Indigenous player to represent Australia in netball when she took to the court against New Zealand in Christchurch in May 1986. As she explains: 'participation in sport was my mother's way of managing 12 children' (Ella-Duncan cited in Herbert 2010)

Ella-Duncan started her netball career at 9 years old playing with La Perouse Netball Club. After making the decision to take netball further, she moved across to Randwick Rugby Netball Club. She represented the club in the under 12 team and continued throughout her teens and early twenties. At 20 years old Ella-Duncan was invited to trial for the Australian Institute of Sport (AIS) Netball Program and became the first Aboriginal person to receive a scholarship into the AIS. She played 18 Tests for Australia, and her career included winning a silver medal at the 1987 Netball World Cup in Glasgow, Scotland.

Like many Indigenous Australians, Ella-Duncan became aware of racism at an early age, 'I did experience racism, some very interesting and subtle forms of racism' (Ella-Duncan cited in Herbert 2010). She explains:

> When I was younger, I was quite oblivious to this issue – I was mainly having fun. As I got a little older and started trying out for representative teams, I never made it onto any of the teams. It didn't bother me at the time because I was quite shy but later, I found out that my sports teacher had been so upset that I had been overlooked. In her mind, it had clearly been racism as I had been the far better player but had been overlooked because I was the only Aboriginal player.
>
> As I got older and worldlier, I encountered not so much direct racism as institutional racism and stereotyping. I had experiences where

> people would say that I had gone 'walkabout'[1] or that I was unreliable but they didn't understand my circumstances, for example that my parents did not drive so I had to catch public transport to get to training and games (Ella-Duncan cited in Walker 2010).

For all her ground-breaking work within the sport of netball, Ella-Duncan was inducted into the NSW and Australian Netball Hall of Fame and awarded the Order of Australia Medal in 1988. She continues to coach netball at the Randwick Netball Association but laments the on-going expectations for her to act as a SRM. 'Even now I'm considered a really strong role model, which is sad really, because I should have been usurped by now' (Ella-Duncan cited in George 2017).

Ella-Duncan has held senior state government and ATSIC positions, was Chair of La Perouse Local Aboriginal Land Council from 2009-2017 and has participated in various high-level review committees. She has worked with Netball Australian to develop a Reconciliation Action Plan, launched in 2015. The Plan was aimed at extending opportunities to grow and thrive to all Aboriginal women and girls. Speaking at the launch, Ella Duncan said: 'We know sport delivers so many benefits, and there is no other demographic in Australia that needs those opportunities more than my Aboriginal and Torres Strait Islander sisters' (Ella-Duncan cited in ALM 2015).

However, the sport of netball continues to struggle in its efforts to understand the experiences of players, coaches, umpires and administrators, and identifying the barriers to greater Aboriginal and Torres Strait Islander participation, and once again Ella-Duncan has been called upon to provided leadership to help the organization deliver change (Monteverde 2020). She describes her intentions:

> I'm really interested in what can we do right now to get things moving and at the same time create an environment that is inclusive of

[1] 'Going walkabout' is a derogative term, used when someone doesn't turn up or is late. It is considered offensive because it implies Aboriginal societies are not as 'advanced' and reliable as European societies.

> all women and girls so that it becomes business as usual. (Ella-Duncan cited in Holmes 2020)

Ella-Duncan remains a rare female Indigenous voice in sports governance. Yet she hopes that the efforts of Netball Australia and its state bodies will eventually yield some Indigenous stars that can usurp her (George 2017).

JEMMA MIMI

Jemma MiMi is a professional netballer in the Australian Suncorp Netball Superleague competition. As the only Indigenous player in the League, she has recently marked her fifth year with the Queensland-based Firebirds franchise. Highlighting the extent of Indigenous women's absence from the sport's high-performance ranks, only two Indigenous women have worn Netball Australia colours—Marcia Ella-Duncan, who made her debut in 1986, and Sharon Finnan-White, who retired in 2000.

Eventually playing in the topflight netball competition, MiMi's earlier sporting pursuits were on the track:

> my Indigenous role model growing up was Cathy Freeman. I thought she was incredible, plus she looked like me. I was also a runner—I did a lot of track, ran the 400m, 200m, did a lot of sprints. She was just inspiring. (MiMi, 2021)[2]

Combined with Cathy Freeman's influence was her mother's own representative netball background in the Queensland Under 21 team. These two inspirational women laid the foundation for MiMi's emergence as a dominant figure on and off the court, 'Mum was a

---

[2] An Australian household name, Cathy Freeman is considered as one of Australia's greatest ever sportspeople. Cathy was the leader for athletics in Australia during the 1990s and at the 2000 Sydney Olympic Games, inspiring thousands of Australians to pursue the sport.

netballer who'd represented Queensland … and she got me into it [netball] just to make new friends because I was quite shy' (MiMi, 2021).

Coinciding with Jemma MiMi's entry to the Netball Superleague, the competition staged its first Indigenous round. The Indigenous round was promoted as an important opportunity to celebrate Indigenous culture and encourage meaningful cultural exchange. With the theme 'Because of her, we can' and focusing on the many Indigenous women who are 'significant role models at community, local, state, and national levels', the Indigenous Round was part of the sport's efforts to provide an inclusive environment for all Australians to participate in and enjoy netball. MiMi's presence in the Superleague soon became a focus for celebration. But cast into the spotlight, her image and profile, including her own recent journey discovering and connecting with her Indigenous cultural heritage, caught her off guard.

> I still don't know very much but I'm learning every day and I want to know more. It helps me now, understanding little things about myself and why I am the way I am. (MiMi 2019)

Despite her visibility in the Superleague's Indigenous round marketing campaign MiMi did not receive court time during the game. Her demotion to the bench was profoundly criticised. Indeed, the ensuing criticism and media reporting further cast MiMi into the media spotlight, 'Being the only Indigenous player, the expectation was to see me on court, and when that didn't happen, it let a lot of people down, unfortunately' (MiMi 2021). The layers of complexity arising from MiMi's absence from the court were further amplified owing to her own interpretation of how Indigenous girls need SRMs in their own image:

> I just hope that young Indigenous girls who've seen me out there on the court can get that belief in their own capability and know that if they've got that love for it and they really want to do it, they can, knowing that there are pathways. (MiMi 2021)

Indigenous scholars such as Oxley (2020, n.p.) interpreted how the Superleague's use of MiMi's image and her cultural background 'reflects the persistent exploitative practices of 'diversity' labour that Aboriginal and/or Torres Strait Islander people are expected to endure in order to participate fully as valued athletes' (Oxley 2020, n.p.). At the same time, Firebird administrators acknowledged that they 'misread community expectations' (Hislop 2020, n.p.). For Jemma MiMi the events exerted unwanted pressure on her to advocate for and represent Indigenous peoples. She expressed feeling a 'worldwide of emotions' along with the hurt and pressure:

> To see the girls, win, I was happy but also sad that I couldn't get on court. I spoke to the girls at the time and our coaches about how I felt and because they just didn't really understand that pressure. (MiMi 2021)

Despite these occurrences MiMi has drawn on her experiences as an opportunity to call for and enable change. Indeed, her voice has been amplified and it has seen her speak of her desire to be an SRM, 'I absolutely love being a part of the program'. Undeniably, her involvement in Netball Queensland's Diamond Spirit Program—a community engagement program that uses netball as a vehicle to engage, empower, and educate Aboriginal and Torres Strait Islander girls in remote and regional communities across Queensland—has been an important and rewarding undertaking.

> It has helped me to grow and own my cultural journey as well as facilitate a safe place for discussions about our rich culture and what they might be learning about at school. (MiMi cited in Ellis 2020)

Criticisms of the 2020 Netball Superleague Indigenous round and MiMi's voice have seen Netball Australia publicly commit to improvements for Indigenous players. In an historic move, 20 of the sport's national, state and territory based, and club bodies have signed a Declaration of Commitment to 'break down the barriers that have prevented Aboriginal and Torres Strait Islander players, coaches, umpires and administrators from flourishing in the sport' (Netball Australia 2020). An unequivocal apology together with a 'true partnership' approach underpinned by the principle of 'trust and mutual respect' has seen the code and sport commit to redressing the barriers confronting Aboriginal and Torres Strait Islander girls and women's full participation in the sport (Netball Australia 2020).

Evonne Goolagong-Cawley

Born in 1951, Wiradjuri woman Evonne Goolagong-Cawley[3] was thc first Aboriginal person to play tennis, and was characterized as the best known and acclaimed Aboriginal athlete in the world (Tatz 1987). Like many successful Indigenous athletes, she is said to have experienced a 'victory over adversity' story. Life started as one of eight children in an Aboriginal family in rural New South Wales. Reflecting on her childhood, Goolagong-Cawley recalls not experiencing overt discrimination. Rather, her family was well-respected in the small outback town of Barellan, where townsfolk were credited with supporting her tennis pursuits raising funds and celebrating her accomplishments. Aged about 10 Goolagong-Cawley was 'adopted' by tennis coach Vic Edwards, who became a powerful influence on her tennis and personal life (Stell 1991). She gained national and worldwide acclaim, winning four Australian singles titles, the Italian, French and South African Opens and was the Wimbledon singles champion in 1971 and 1980. Goolagong-Cawley was named Female Athlete and Australian of the Year in 1971. Later she became the chief Aboriginal representative of the 2000 Sydney Olympic Games.

The end of the 1960s was a time when there was a feeling of atonement about Australian Aboriginal people, and for a time, Goolagong-Cawley's abstinence from Aboriginal affairs and politics

---

[3] Evonne Goolagong married Roger Cawley on 19 June 1975 and adopted the name Evonne Goolagong Cawley.

positively shaped her interactions with an 'adoring public' (Tatz 1995, p. 276). While she remained outside Aboriginal affairs and politics, (most) people 'just loved her' (Tatz 1995, p. 276). However, her visit to South Africa in 1971 sparked controversy. While there, she received preferential treatment as if she were white, and in Australia, a huge media storm erupted. Condemned for insulting her own people for entertaining racists with her tennis prowess, media pressed her for comments on South Africa's refusal of a visa for Arthur Ashe, and activist Charles Perkins reproached her for not using her prestige of behalf of Aboriginal people. The ultimate insult came when she was accused of being 'more white' than Aboriginal (Hargreaves 2000). Goolagong-Cawley became the uncomfortable subject of national debate, caught between the powerful, colonial elites and those of the national and international Aboriginal communities, who continued to criticize her for doing nothing about Aboriginal affairs, failing to speak out on land rights and racial issues and for being insulated from the problems of most Aboriginal women (Stell 1991).

After exploring the politics of race in apartheid South Africa, Goolagong-Cawley turned to researching her family history. Previously unrecognized, she became keenly aware of the discrimination her family experienced. She promoted a book on Aboriginal oral history because, she claimed, 'I'm just sort of proud that I am Aboriginal, and this is the first book I've seen that has Aborigines speaking out for themselves' (Goolagong-Cawley cited in Tatz 1995, p. 64). The fact that she was a founding member of the National Aboriginal Sports Foundation and became open about her own Aboriginality re-established her credibility—for a time—as a SRM and as a figurehead for unity during the Sydney 2000 proceedings. However, once again she remained silent about the ways in which Sydney 2000 became a platform for Aboriginal protest and politics aimed to stir and embarrass state and national governments (Hargreaves 2000). Not surprisingly, the interpretation was implicit—as support for those in positions of power (Hargreaves 2000), once again clearly not an embodiment of the elements most dear to Indigenous society (Maguire 2009).

Goolagong-Cawley appears to have always considered herself a SRM and example rather than a political spokesperson. Playing tennis, she could represent Aboriginal people at the same time as she represented Australia, and she could fulfil such a representative role without being overtly political (Fox 2011). Tennis gave her a voice through which she could play this role. After all, she said, “If I hadn’t become a champion, who would listen to me now?” (Goolagong-Cawley and Jarratt 1993, p. 12).

Ashleigh Barty

In 2021, 25-year-old Queenslander, Ashleigh (Ash) Barty was ranked No. 1 in singles by the Women’s Tennis Association (WTA). She is a top 20 player in doubles, having achieved a career-high ranking of No. 5 in the world. Barty has won eight singles titles and ten doubles titles on the WTA Tour, including Grand Slam singles titles at the 2019 French Open and Wimbledon in 2021, and one Grand Slam doubles title at the 2018 US Open. She is the reigning champion in singles at the WTA Finals.

Ash Barty grew up in Springfield, in Queensland, Australia. Her father, Robert is a member of the Ngarigo people from southern NSW and north-eastern Victoria, and her mother, Josie, is the daughter of English immigrants. Barty has focused on strengthening the identity, values and sense of wider community of Indigenous Australians since gaining the spotlight. Her career rise has been meteoric, to say the least. Perhaps tellingly, Barty was one of the very few to have a renowned female Indigenous SRM growing up—Evonne Goolagong-Cawley.

> Evonne has absolutely created the pathway, not just for Indigenous boys and girls, but kids across the nation. … She is just such a special person, and I’m incredibly lucky to share heritage with her. That is a very special part of me that I’m extremely proud of, and I know she is as well. (Barty, cited in Lilly 2019)

Barty's career rise has been meteoric. Since gaining the spotlight she has focused on strengthening the identity, values, and sense of wider community of Indigenous Australians. Reflecting further on her relationship and shared cultural history with Goolagong-Cawley, Barty explains:

> Deep down, we are friends … most importantly, we are family. That is something not many people can say, and we share that really special heritage, which is probably the most special thing about our relationship' (Barty cited in Walsh 2019)

Barty appears to be benefitting from the experiences of Indigenous women before her, perhaps learning from their mistakes in the public arena. She seems careful not to become enmeshed in political or sporting controversies and seems wary of passing judgement on fellow players (Pierik 2019). However, she raised some eyebrows when she deviated from her normal course by bringing her baby niece to her post-match press conference after her 2020 Australian Open semifinal loss. Barty was called out by former Australian tennis great Mark Woodforde for—in his eyes—using a young child as a shield to deflect the tough questions that all tennis players face when they experience a difficult loss. 'As number one player in the world, the press want to know when you lose a match, why you've lost a match, they want you to bear your soul' Woodforde said (cited in Glover 2020).

Nevertheless, this carefully-constructed image is reaping benefits, with Barty lauded as the 'hero that Australian tennis needed' (Kovalchik 2019). Presently her on-court earnings are about $18,798,304, from singles and doubles tennis on the WTA Tour. In 2020 she was ranked as the third-highest paid female athlete in the world. She earned $13.1 million, with $10.1 million coming in prize money (Tennis Australia 2020).

Barty continues to make a name for herself. In the same way that Goolagong-Cawley was a huge mentor for Barty, she hopes to be a mentor for youths in the Aboriginal community. She says her heritage is important to her and refers to her olive complexion and 'squished nose', saying 'I just think it's important to do the best I can to be a good role model (Barty, cited in Marshall 2019).' Barty appears to be doing just that and was appointed National Indigenous Tennis Ambassador in 2018.

> This annual National Indigenous Tennis Carnival will be an amazing event, for not only tennis across Australia but especially Indigenous tennis. To bring all of the kids together to give them an opportunity to showcase what they're capable of. (Barty, cited in Gunawardana 2020b)

Discussion

The preceding section presented vignettes of six Indigenous Australian sportswomen and their careers. The narratives briefly explored how Indigenous women's SRM status have been constructed, navigated, and contested in complex and paradoxical ways, and often between cultures. The research questions explored were:

1. What are the perceived roles and functions of female Indigenous SRMs?
2. How do Meier's (2015) theoretical models help to provide an understanding of the contested, emerging, and changeable nature of these sportswomen as SRMs?

Indigenous Australian sportswomen appear highly motivated and focused individuals who have the opportunity to be seen as exemplars for other Indigenous women to enter sport with a strong sense of self (Stronach 2013). While not all athletes would necessarily have the motivations, skills or values to aspire to positions of 'custodians of virtue', what has been most evident in the stories has been the determined effort of the women to utilize the opportunities provided for them by sport to grasp, albeit in different ways and at different times, the SRM persona. It is apparent that, 'Aboriginal women can't move through the world without the weight of the politics around us'(James cited in O'Shea, Stronach, and Maxwell 2020). We have seen how Indigenous Australian sportswomen are unavoidably caught up in the politics of Aboriginality and the dilemma of identity, and frequently characterized as perpetuating a story of 'victory over adversity'. They are habitually described in the mainstream (white) Australian media as 'black', 'colored', or 'Aboriginal'. Each woman who features in this chapter has, at times and in varying ways, experienced racism and discrimination. Each of them has navigated their representation in different ways tempered by their political position on Indigenous or social issues.

Meier's (2015) nine functions are clearly recognizable within the cohort examined. Certainly, most of the athletes can be seen to have used—some more purposefully than others—their sporting achievements to develop a profile enabling them to influence and support other Indigenous people. They displayed and clearly articulated a special set of personal values: pride in their Indigenous heritage, unique kinship and community obligations, along with a commitment to support disadvantaged Indigenous people, be it formally or informally. The obligation to 'give back' to family and community was the 'natural order' of Indigenous sportswomen. Indigenous Australian sportswomen are highly motivated and focused individuals who have the opportunity to be seen as exemplars for other Indigenous women to enter sport with a strong sense of self (Stronach 2013). This is not dissimilar to the experiences of other marginalized women in Australia, for example Mecca Laa Laa, who in 2005, became the first Muslim woman surf lifesaver. In doing she was an inspiration for others and was keen to 'give back' to her community and empower other Muslim women to participate in sporting activities (Maxwell 2012).

While not all Indigenous athletes would necessarily have the motivations, skills, or values to aspire to positions of 'custodians of virtue', what has been most evident has been the determination of the women to leverage the opportunities provided for them by sport to develop an athletic career and then utilize their athletic success to influence and inspire other Indigenous people—that is as an SRM.

The idea of 'giving back' to community and a commitment to support disadvantaged Indigenous people is a strong desire of most, if not all the profiled Indigenous sportswomen. However, these efforts are not without complexity and challenge. Working in remote and challenged Indigenous communities has noble intentions, but the practicality of turning such activity into a career is fraught with difficulties, and such a commitment may very well be to the detriment to the economic well-being of retired athletes themselves (Stronach, Adair, and Taylor 2014). Few community support roles generate much (or indeed any) income, and there is little prospect, from within that environment, for further professional development. For many former athletes, community support work remains philanthropic and voluntary. However, if Indigenous sportswomen are provided with appropriate leadership and mentoring skills, such as those provided by some national sporting organisations including Tennis Australia and Cricket Australia, these efforts can also be socio-culturally virtuous and 'life-changing'. Leadership training is valuable and worthy preparation with many potential transferabilities (Stronach, Adair, and Taylor 2014). Vitally important in such programs would be cultural education sessions (Gunawardana 2020a).

We also see a fluidity—even a volatility—in the SRM persona that is illustrated in Meier's (2015) continuum, illustrated in Figure 1. Each of the three contemporary sportswomen discusses the influence of their predecessors i.e., other Indigenous SRMs. In line with the continuum we see the three women who have retired from sport exerting considerable influence as Type 1 SRMs. Faith Thomas continues to vocalise her concerns around women's cricket, and Evonne Goolagong-Cawley remains extremely active through her charitable Foundation in supporting young Indigenous girls and boys. Despite Marcia Ella-Duncan's discomfort that she is still expected to inspire Indigenous netballers, she continues in her coaching roles at high performance levels, as a Type 2 SRM. The younger women have reflected on the inspiration they have drawn from Type 3 SRMs. For example, Jemma MiMi has discussed the role Cathy Freeman played in her life, Ashleigh Gardner has recognized Faith Thomas's pioneering sporting prowess, and Ashleigh Barty continues to be motivated by Evonne Goolagong-Cawley in both her personal and sporting lives. Owing to their Indigeneity these two women today identify as family.

According to Maguire (2009, 1261), 'If a sportsperson wants to achieve heroic status, he or she has to 'embod[y] the elements that a society holds most dear'. Several of the women have illustrated how at times, they oscillated between deviance and hero status, 'embodying the elements that a society holds most dear'—depending on which society they are trying to appease. For example, Faith Thomas became a culturally relevant figure who appears to embody the elements that her society holds most dear. Along with racism and discrimination in 1930s Australian society, Faith Thomas experienced fundamental disparities in the participation, profile and power of men in cricket as opposed to women, at a time when cricketing women had little voice and even less decision-making power (Stronach and Adair 2009). Perhaps unsurprisingly, it has been Faith Thomas, the oldest of the six sportswomen, to call out and challenge what she sees as gender inequity in women's sport.

The two tennis players, Goolagong-Cawley and Barty have oscillated between deviance and hero status. Evonne Goolagong-Cawley was the 'darling of white society' but lost credibility with Aboriginal people when she appeared to support the South African apartheid movement. Ashleigh Barty was castigated for taking a baby to a press conference—ostensibly to shield herself from criticism over her performance. Arguably, SRMs are never just famous or heroic in isolation—they are socially constructed (Maguire 2009), and continuously negotiate their SRM identities. This constructionist approach also underpins the fluidity of their SRM roles. Rather than agreed and enduring, the women's identities are contested, emerging and changeable. This is what we see as a paradox of identity for these women. Both Goolagong-Cawley and Barty were ultimately and retrospectively legitimized, and 'forgiven' due, it seems, to their sporting success (Wrench and Garrett 2018).

Jemma MiMi's experiences demonstrate how Indigenous women's presence is simultaneously valued and devalued. While her presence as the only Indigenous professional netballer at the Superleague's Indigenous Round was celebrated, her voice and experiences were not. The deep personal costs and pressures placed on her, especially as a young woman, are a significant concern. The parallels between her experiences and those of Evonne Goolagong-Cawley in terms of the profound and lofty expectations placed on their shoulders to advocate for Indigenous Australians at such a young age demonstrate how little has changed or has been learnt. Indeed, Marcia Ella-Duncan's frustrations at being considered an SRM some 30 years since her retirement from representative netball illustrate the slowness and costs associated with advocating and advancing change. Notwithstanding the personal costs, and pressures, we can see how taken-for-granted racialized practices, discourses and norms can be challenged. When Indigenous women's voices and experiences are heard through a process of deep and respectful listening, a more meaningful pathway to change can be enabled.

Our study has identified a further function of female Indigenous SRMs. We conceptualize this function as *cultural maintenance*. The following discussion is offered to justify this contention. In Indigenous communities, sport has long been an integral component of everyday life (Tatz 2009). Generally, they were gendered, age-related, and intimately connected to Aboriginal family kinship and culture (Phillips and Osmond 2018). Sport now provides a social space for Indigenous women to connect to cultural practices, languages, and ways of being and knowing. This is both a means of participating in cultural activity and a way to maintain culture (Stronach, Maxwell, and Taylor 2015). Indeed, in previous research, female Indigenous interviewees described themselves as 'keepers of the culture' (Gymea, cited in Stronach, Maxwell, and Taylor 2015, 14). The women involved in the current research seized the opportunities that sport enabled them to maintain culture. For Goolagong-Cawley, Barty, MiMi, and Gardner, maintenance of their culture occurred alongside their own journeys of cultural discovery. In addition, this deeper knowledge further equipped them with the knowledge and passion to advocate on behalf of their people.

CONCLUSION

This analysis of six Indigenous Australian sportswomen's biographies enables a deeper understanding of the unique platform provided by sport for the women to amplify their voices and support other Indigenous people. The nine SRM functions of participation, leadership, advocacy, challenging gender stereotypes, inspiration, ethics, safeguarding and prevention, media and corporates, and giving back (Meier 2015) provide a useful framework for this analysis. Our work also identifies a tenth function of Indigenous SRMs, that of cultural maintenance, which appears to have the potential a give further voice to female Indigenous athletes and achieve wider societal influence.

Further research is needed to untangle the complexities and fluidity of female Indigenous Australian SRMs in the evolving worlds of professional and community sport. We acknowledge that this study was limited by the women's involvement in elite level sports. The contemporary Indigenous sportswomen selected all compete—or did compete—professionally and at the highest level of their sport. Future research exploring Indigenous women participating as players, coaches and officials at the community level of sport could provide some useful insights in the future.

That Indigenous Australian sportswomen continue to inspire the next generation has been shown to be especially true. Valuing these women's voices, lived experiences, interpretations and desires challenges the legitimacy of Anglo western ways of knowing and being. Female Indigenous Australian SRMs can be powerful role models for us all.

References

Primary Sources

Gardner, Ashleigh. (2017-2021). *Facebook posts and Twitter feeds.*

MiMi, Jemma. (2017-2021). *Facebook posts and Twitter feeds.*

Secondary Sources

Adair, Daryl. 2015. Athletes of influence? The role model refrain in sport *The Conversation*.

ALM. 2015. Netball Australia launches inaugural Reconciliation Action Plan. *Australasian Leisure Management News*.

Ashleigh Gardner Foundation. 2021. "Ashleigh Gardner Foundation." Ashleigh Gardner Foundation.

Australian Bureau of Statistics. 2016. "Census: Aboriginal and Torres Strait Islander population." *ABS.* http://www.abs.gov.au/ausstats/abs@.nsf/mediareleasesbyReleaseDate/02D50FAA9987D6B7CA25814800087E03?OpenDocument.

Australian Institute of Health and Welfare. 2015. *The health and welfare of Australia's Aboriginal and Torres Strait Islander peoples Cat. No. IHW 147*. Canberra: AIHW.

Burney, Linda. 2019. "Behind the scenes, Ashleigh Barty has been giving back." *The Sydney Morning Herald*. https://www.smh.com.au/sport/tennis/behind-the-scenes-ashleigh-barty-has-been-giving-back-20190609-p51vzr.html.

Clarey, Christopher. 2000. "Running Toward, and From, History " *The New York Times*, 21 March. https://archive.nytimes.com/www.nytimes.com/learning/students/pop/032100oly-freeman.html.

De Croock, Stephanie, Veerle De Bosscher, and Maarten van Bottenburg. 2012. "The inspirational function of role models for sport participation and development." *20th Conference of the European Association for Sport Management*, Aalborg, Denmark de Leeuw, S, M. Greenwood, and M Farrales. 2021. "Indigeneity and wellness: Critically understanding the health of Indigenous peoples and communities." In *Routledge International Handbook of Critical Issues in Health and Illness*, 197-208. London: Routledge.

Dix, S, I Phau, and S Pougnet. 2010. "Bend it like Beckham": the influence of sports celebrities on young adult consumers." *Young Consumers* 11 (1): 36–46.

Ellis, Liz. 2020. The Mi Mi debacle can't happen again. *The Sydney Morning Herald*.

Ferguson, Leah, Gillian B Epp, Kellie Wuttunee, Matthew Dunn, Tara-Leigh McHugh, and M. Louise Humbert. 2019. "It's more than just performing well in your sport. It's also about being healthy physically, mentally, emotionally, and spiritually': Indigenous women athletes' meanings and experiences of flourishing in sport." *Qualitative Research in Sport, Exercise and Health* 11 (1). doi: DOI: 10.1080/2159676X.2018.1458332.

Fox, Karen. 2011. "Representing Difference, 1950-2000." In *Māori and Aboriginal Women in the Public Eye*, edited by Karen Fox, 49-75. Canberra: ANU Press.

George, Eric. 2017. Why Marcia Ella-Duncan wishes she wasn't a role model anymore. *The Weekend Australian*.

Glover, Ben. 2020. Australian tennis legend Mark Woodforde calls out Ash Barty's press conference stunt. *Wide World of Sports*.

Goodall, Heather. 1995. "Assimilation Begins in the Home: The State and Aboriginal Women's Work as Mothers in New South Wales, 1900s to 1960s." *Labour History* 69 (1):89-95.

Goolagong-Cawley, E, and P Jarratt. 1993. *Home! The Evonne Goolagong Story*. East Roseville: Simon and Schuster.

Gray, Caitlin, Rona Macniven, and Neil Thomson. 2013. *Review of physical activity among Indigenous people.* Canberra: Australian Indigenous Health InfoNet.

Green, Amy. 2019. "Another feather in Faith Thomas' baggy green." *Moree Champion* https://www.moreechampion.com.au/story/6209309/another-feather-in-faith-thomas-baggy-green/.

Grix, Jonathan, and Fiona Carmichael. 2012. "Why do governments invest in elite sport? A polemic." *International Journal of Sport Policy and Politics* 4 (1):73-90.

Gunawardana, Tash. 2020a. "AFLW illustrates importance of Indigenous role models." *Siren: A women in sport collective*. https://sirensport.com.au/aussie-rules/aflw/aflw-illustrates-importance-of-indigenous-role-models/.

Gunawardana, Tash 2020b. The rise of Barty and the importance of Indigenous role models. *The Women's Game*.

Hargreaves, Jennifer. 2000. *Heroines of Sport: The Politics of Difference and Identity*. London and New York: Routledge.

Hayhurst, Lyndsay, Audrey Giles, and Jan Wright. 2016. "The benefits and challenges of girl-focused Indigenous SDP programs in Australia and Canada." In *Beyond Sport for Development and Peace: Transnational perspectives on theory, policy and practice*, edited by L.N.C Hayhurst, T Kay and M Chawansky, 111-127. Abingdon, United Kingdom: Routledge.

Herbert, Bronwyn. 2010. Sporting codes put on notice over racism. *AM*.

Hislop, Madeline. 2020. Firebirds coach says she 'misread community expectations' by sidelining Jemma Mi Mi during Super Netball's Indigenous Round. *Women's Agenda*.

Holmes, Tracey. 2020. Netball's Indigenous Diamonds call for immediate action on diversity; Netball Queensland commits to change. *ABC News*.

Ishigami, Hideaki. 2019. *Estimating the impact of the 2011 FIFA Women's World Cup on Japanese adolescent girls: a causal analysis of sports role models*. 11 (3):503-519.

Jackson, R 2016. Aboriginal cricket pioneer Faith Thomas: 'I'm still the fastest woman bowler ever'. *The Guardian*.

Kovalchik, Stephanie. 2019. The numbers game: how Ash Barty became the world's best female tennis player *The Conversation*.

Krieken, R. V. 1999. "The 'Stolen Generations' and cultural genocide: The forced removal of Australian Indigenous children from their families and its implications for the sociology of childhood." *Childhood* 6 (3):297-311.

Lilly, Alex. 2019. Australian Open 2019: Who is tennis superstar Ash Barty? *The Australian Women's Weekly*.

Lines, Gill. 2001. "Villains, fools or heroes? Sports stars as role models for young people." *Leisure Studies* 20 (4):285-303.

Maguire, Joseph. 2009. "The Social Construction and Impact of Champions." *Sport in Society* 12: (9: Special Issue: The Social Impact of Sport):1250–1264.

Mallett, Ashley. 2018. *The Boys from St Francis: Stories of the remarkable Aboriginal activists* Mile End: Wakefield Press.

Marshall, Konrad. 2019. Second Serve. *The Sydney Morning Herald*.

Mason, C, and J Koehli. 2012. "Barriers to Physical Activity for Aboriginal Youth: Implications for Community Health, Policy, and Culture." *Pimatisiwin: A Journal of Aboriginal and Indigenous Community Health* 10 (1):97-107.

Maxwell, Hazel. 2012. *An exploration of social inclusion in Australian community sport: the case of Muslim women*. PhD, UTS.

Maxwell, Hazel, Michelle O'Shea, Megan Stronach, and Sonya Pearce. 2019. "Empowerment through digital health trackers: an exploration of Indigenous Australian women and physical activity in leisure settings." *Annals of Leisure Research*:1-18. doi: 10.1080/11745398.2019.1674677.

Maxwell, Hazel, Megan Stronach, Daryl Adair, and Sonya Pearce. 2017. "Indigenous Australian women and sport: Findings and recommendations from a parliamentary inquiry." *Sport in Society (Online)*:1-29. doi: 10.1080/17430437.2017.1284802.

Meier, Marianne. 2015. "The value of female sporting role models." *Sport in Society* 18 (8):968-982.

Midgley, C, G DeBues-Stafford, P Lockwood, and S Thai. 2021. "She needs to see it to be it: The importance of same-gender athletic role models." *Sex Roles*:1-19.

Monga, Sidharth 2019. Faith Thomas is the Aussie legend you haven't heard of. *The Cricket Monthly*.

Monteverde, Marco 2020. Netball: Officials vow to address lack of indigenous representation at all levels after Queensland Firebird Jemma Mi Mi's indigenous round snub raised historical issues. *News.com.au.*

Netball Australia. 2020. *Our commitment to listen, learn and change.* accessed 20 February. https://netball.com.au/news/our-commitment-listen-learn-and-change.

Nicholson, Rowan. 2021. Yes, this continent was invaded in 1788 – an international law expert explain. *The Conversation.*

O'Shea, Michelle, Megan Stronach, and Hazel Maxwell. 2020. More than a tennis story: Sunshine Super Girl is challenging inequities and enabling inclusive possibilities. *SirenSport.*

O'Shea, Michelle, Hazel Maxwell, and Megan Stronach. 2020. "Reconciliatory Action and the Gold Coast Commonwealth Games: Inclusion for Indigenous Australian women?" *Sporting Traditions* 37 (2):71-91.

Oxley, Robyn. 2020. OPINION: Indigenous Round is not a marketing strategy, repeat after me *NITV Latest news.*

Parker, Lesley. 2015. *To be or not to be: sports role models.*

Phillips, Murray, and Gary Osmond. 2018. "Australian Indigenous Sport Historiography: A Review." *Kinesiology Review* 7 (2):193-198.

Pierik, Jon. 2019. Barty on a roll and ready to be a role model. *The Sydney Mornng Herald.*

Reiner, M, C Niermann, D Jekauc, and A Woll. 2013. "Long term health benefits of physical activity - a systemic review." *BMC Public Health* 13:1-9.

Rowley, K.G, M Daniel, K Skinner, M Skinner, G.A White, and K O'Dea. 2000. "Effectiveness of a community-directed 'healthy lifestyle' program in a remote Australian aboriginal community " *Aust N Z J Public Health* 24 (2):136-44.

Stell, Marion. 1991. *Half the Race: A History of Australian Women in Sport.* North Ryde: Collins.

Stronach, Megan 2013. 'Game over': Indigenous athletes transitioning out of sport. *Sport Business Insider.*

Stronach, Megan, and Daryl Adair. 2009. "'Brave new world' or 'sticky wicket'? Women, management and organizational power in Cricket Australia." *Sport in Society: Cultures, Commerce, Media, Politics* 12 (7):910-932.

Stronach, Megan, Daryl Adair, and Tracy Taylor. 2014. "'Game over': Indigenous Australian sportsmen and athletic retirement." *Australian Aboriginal Studies* 2:40-59.

Stronach, Megan, Hazel Maxwell, and Sonya Pearce. 2018. "Indigenous Australian women promoting health through sport." *Sport Management Review*. doi: https://doi.org/10.1016/j.smr.2018.04.007.

Stronach, Megan, Hazel Maxwell, and Tracey Taylor. 2015. "'Sistas' and Aunties: Sport, Physical Activity and Indigenous Australian Women." *Annals of Leisure Research*:1-20. doi: 10.1080/11745398.2015.1051067.

Stronach, Megan, and Michelle O'Shea. 2021. "Learning, understanding and valuing Indigenous peoples' leisure." *Annals of Leisure Research* 24 (1):1-5. doi: DOI: 10.1080/11745398.2021.1881709

Tatz, Colin. 1987. *Aborigines in Sport*. Sydney: Australian Society for Sports History.

Tatz, Colin. 1995. *Obstacle race: Aborigines in sport*. Kensington: NSW University Press.

Tatz, Colin. 2009. "The Meaning of Life Is … Sport." *The Sydney Morning Herald*, 12 December, 34.

Tennis Australia. 2020. Barty named one of the world's highest-paid female athletes. *News*.

UN. 2007. *Women, Gender Equality and Sport: Women 2000 and beyond.* New York: United Nations, Division for Advancement of Women, Department of Economic and Social Affairs.

Walker, Ashley. 2010. An Interview with Marcia Ella-Duncan. *Indigenous Law Bulletin*.

Walsh, Courtney. 2019. 'She paved the way' the bond between Ash Barty and Evonne Goolagong Cawley goes far beyond tennis. *The Weekend Australian Magazine*.

Walsh, Liz. 2020. Ashleigh Gardner and Australian women's cricket teammates flying flag to end racism on home front. *The Advertiser*.

Wrench, A, and R Garrett. 2018. "Constructions of Australia's sportswomen: 'Race','whiteness' and contemporary media." *Sport, Education and Society* 23 (8):748-760.

BIOGRAPHICAL SKETCHES

Megan Stronach

Affiliation: University Technology Sydney

Education: BA, BN, M. Sport Mgt, PhD

Research and Professional Experience:

2018 – 2021	Research Fellow	University of Technology Sydney
2020 – current	Lecturer	University of Tasmania
2014 – 2021	Researcher	University of Tasmania

Professional Appointments:

- Executive Committee, Australian Society of Sports Historians
- Sport Management Association of Australia and New Zealand

Publications from the Last 3 Years:

1. Stronach, Megan. 2018. Cultural Change or An Uneasy Truce? Forestry and Tourism in Geeveston, Southern Tasmania. *Tasmanian Historical Studies Journal 22:*55-71.
2. Stronach, Megan, Daryl Adair, and Hazel Maxwell. 2019. "'Djabooly-djabooly: why don't they swim?': the ebb and flow of water in the lives of Australian Aboriginal women." *Annals of Leisure Research* 22:286-304.

3. Stronach, Megan, Hazel Maxwell, and Sonya Pearce. 2019. "Indigenous Australian women promoting health through sport." *Sport Management Review* 22:5-20.
4. Stronach, Megan and Daryl Adair. 2019. Hidden women of history: Wauba Debar, an Indigenous swimmer from Tasmania who saved her captors. *The Conversation*, 30 December 2019.
5. O'Shea, Michelle and Megan Stronach, 2019. For many, a pool swim is an Australian birthright. Let's make it easier for solo parents to claim it. *The Conversation*, 30 December 2019.
6. O'Shea, Michelle, Hazel Maxwell, and Megan Stronach, and Sonya Pearce. 2020. Sport can be an important part of Aboriginal culture for women–but many barriers remain. *The Conversation*, 23 January 2020.
7. O'Shea, Michelle, Hazel Maxwell, and Megan Stronach. 2020. Why should my child take swimming lessons? And what do they need to know? *The Conversation*, 7 February 2020.
8. Stronach, Megan and Daryl Adair. 2020. Swimming for their lives: *palawa* women of *lutruwita* (Van Diemen's Land). *Sporting Traditions 37*(2):47-70.
9. O'Shea, Michelle, Hazel Maxwell, and Megan Stronach. 2020 "Reconciliatory action and the Gold Coast Commonwealth Games: Inclusion for Indigenous Australian women?" *Sporting Traditions* 37(2):71-91.
10. Stronach, Megan and Hazel Maxwell. (2020). Developing Sport for Indigenous Women and Girls. In *Developing Sport for Women and Girls,* edited by Emma Sherry, and Katie Rowe, 95-109. London: Routledge.
11. Maxwell, Hazel and Megan Stronach. 2020. "Developing sport for culturally and linguistically diverse women and girls." In *Developing Sport for Women and Girls*, edited by Emma Sherry, and Katie Rowe, 83-94. London: Routledge.
12. O'Shea, Michelle, Megan Stronach, and Hazel Maxwell. 2020. As the bushfire smoke clears sport can be a social anchor, ON LINE *Opinion,* 3 February 2020.

13. O'Shea, Michelle, Megan Stronach, and Hazel Maxwell. 2020. Public pools for all Australians, *Australasian Leisure Management* (137), pp. 48-51.
14. O'Shea, Michelle, Megan Stronach, and Hazel Maxwell. 2020. *Taking back the beach*, 22 May 2020. Open Forum, https://www.openforum.com.au/taking-back-the-beach/
15. O'Shea, Michelle, Megan Stronach, and Hazel Maxwell. 2020. *It's a RAP for indigenous women: Reconciliatory action and the Commonwealth Games*, 3 June 2020. Open Forum, https://www.openforum.com.au/its-a-rap-for-indigenous-women-reconciliatory-action-and-the-commonwealth-games/
16. O'Shea, Michelle, Daryl Adair, Hazel Maxwell, and Megan Stronach. 2020. The Olympics strive for political neutrality. So, how will they deal with surging athlete activism? 18 September 2020. *The Conversation*, https://theconversation.com/ the-olympics-strive-for-political-neutrality-so-how-will-they-deal-with-surging-athlete-activism-144951
17. Darcy, Simon, Jock Collins, and Megan Stronach. 2020. *Opinion: Entrepreneurial spirit built of necessity for people with disability.* 9 November 2020.The Sydney Morning Herald,
18. https://www.smh.com.au/business/workplace/entrepreneurial-spirit-built-of-necessity-for-people-with-disability-20201102-p56at8.html
19. O'Shea, Michelle, Megan Stronach, and Hazel Maxwell. 2020. *More than a tennis story: Sunshine Super Girl is challenging inequities and enabling inclusive possibilities.* 17 November 2020. Siren, https://sirensport.com.au/tennis/more-than-a-tennis-story-sunshine-super-girl-is-challenging-inequities-and-enabling-inclusive-possibilities/
20. O'Shea, Michelle, Hazel Maxwell, and Megan Stronach. 2021. The open Australian beach is a myth: not everyone can access these spaces equally. 21 January 2021. *The Conversation*, https://theconversation.com/the-open-australian-beach-is-a-myth-not-everyone-can-access-these-spaces-equally-153378.

21. Maxwell, Hazel, Michelle O'Shea, Megan Stronach, and Sonya Pearce. 2021. "Empowerment through digital health trackers: An exploration of Indigenous Australian women and physical activity in leisure settings." *Annals of Leisure Research* (24) 1:150-167.
22. Stronach, Megan and Michelle O'Shea. 2021. 'Learning, understanding and valuing Indigenous peoples' leisure', *Annals of Leisure Research*, (24)1:1-5.
23. Stronach, Megan. 2021. 'Time's Up! Indigenous Australian sportsmen and athlete transitions'. In *Athlete Transitions in*
24. *Sport: Experiences in Elite Sport.* Edited by Deborah Agnew, 145-157. London: Routledge.

Hazel Maxwell

Affiliation: University of Tasmania

Education: BA(Hons), MA, PhD

Research and Professional Experience:

2018 – ongoing Senior Lecturer	University of Tasmania
2015 – 2017 Lecturer	University of Tasmania
2007 – 2015 Researcher	University of Technology, Sydney 2007 - 2015

Professional Appointments: Australia and New Zealand Leisure Studies Association

Publications from the Last 3 Years:

1. Darcy, Simon, Hilary Yerbury, and Hazel Maxwell. 2019. "Disability citizenship and digital capital: the case of engagement

with a social enterprise telco." *Information, Communication & Society* 22:538-553.

2. Darcy, Simon, Hazel Maxwell, Simone Grabowski, and Jenny Onyx. 2019. "Artistic impact: From casual and serious leisure to professional career development in disability arts." *Leisure Sciences* Accessed August 25, 2021. doi.org/10.1080/01490400.2019.1613461-20.
3. Harris, Joanna, Kenneth Walsh, Hazel Maxwell, and Susan Dodds. 2019. "Emotional touchpoints; the feelings nurses have about explaining multi-resistant organisms to colonised patients." *Infection, Disease & Health* 25:113-123.
4. Lewis, Gemma K., Hazel Maxwell, and Clayton J. Hawkins. 2019. "Leisure as an agent of social change: special issue introduction." *Annals of Leisure Research.* Accessed August 25, 2021. doi.org/10.1080/11745398.2019.1586308.
5. Maxwell, Hazel, Michelle O'Shea, Megan Stronach, and Sonya Pearce. 2021. "Empowerment through digital health trackers: An exploration of Indigenous Australian women and physical activity in leisure settings." *Annals of Leisure Research* 24:150-167.
6. Maxwell, Hazel, and Megan Stronach. 2020. "Developing sport for culturally and linguistically diverse women and girls." In *Developing Sport for Women and Girls*, edited by Emma Sherry, and Katie Rowe, 83-94. London: Routledge.
7. Maxwell, Hazel, Marguerite Bramble, Sarah J. Prior, Anne Heath, Nicole S. Reeves, Annette Marlow, Steve Campbell, and Douglass J. Doherty. 2021. "Staff experiences of a reablement approach to care for older people in a regional Australian community: A qualitative study." *Health & Social Care in the Community* 29:685-693.
8. O'Shea, Michelle, Hazel Maxwell, and Megan Stronach. 2020 "Reconciliatory action and the gold coast commonwealth games: Inclusion for indigenous Australian women?" *Sporting Traditions* 37:71-91.

9. Peel, Nicole, Hazel Maxwell, and Richard McGrath. 2021. "Leisure and health: conjoined and contested concepts." *Annals of Leisure Research* 24:295-309.
10. Phipps, Monique, Lisa Dalton, Hazel Maxwell, and Michelle Cleary. 2019. "Women and homelessness, a complex multidimensional issue: Findings from a scoping review." *Journal of Social Distress and the Homeless* 28: 1-13.
11. Phipps, Monique, Lisa Dalton, Hazel Maxwell, and Michelle Cleary. 2021. "Combining self-determination theory and photo-elicitation to understand the experiences of homeless women." *Issues in Mental Health Nursing* 42:164-171.
12. Phipps, Monique, Lisa Dalton, Hazel Maxwell, and Michelle Cleary. 2021. "A qualitative exploration of women's resilience in the face of homelessness." *Journal of Community Psychology*. Accessed August 25, 2021. doi.org/10.1002/jcop.22574.
13. Prior, Sarah J., Anne Heath, Nicole S. Reeves, Steven J. Campbell, Hazel Maxwell, Marguerite Bramble, Annette Marlow, and Douglass Doherty. 2021. "Determining readiness for a reablement approach to care in Australia: Development of a pre-employment questionnaire." *Health & Social Care in the Community* 29:685-693.
14. Stronach, Megan, Hazel Maxwell, and Sonya Pearce. 2019. "Indigenous Australian women promoting health through sport." *Sport Management Review* 22:5-20.
15. Stronach, Megan, Daryl Adair, and Hazel Maxwell. 2019. "'Djabooly-djabooly: why don't they swim?': the ebb and flow of water in the lives of Australian Aboriginal women." *Annals of Leisure Research* 22:286-304.
16. Stronach, Megan, and Hazel Maxwell. 2020. "Developing sport for Indigenous women and girls." In *Developing Sport for Women and Girls*, edited by Emma Sherry, and Katie Rowe, 94-109. London: Routledge.

17. Young, Janette, Hazel Maxwell, and Nicole Peel. 2021. "Leisure meets health: important intersections and alternative discourses." *Annals of Leisure Research* 24:275-282.

Michelle O'Shea

Affiliation: University of Western Sydney

Education: BA(Hons), PhD

Research and Professional Experience:

2018 – ongoing Senior Lecturer	Western Sydney University
2006 – 2017 Lecturer	Western Sydney University
2002 – 2006 Researcher	University of Technology, Sydney

Publications from the Last 3 Years:

1. Duarte Alonso, Abel, Seng Kiat Kok, and Michelle O'Shea.2020. Perceived contributory leisure in the context of hobby beekeeping: a multi-country comparison. *Leisure Studies* 40: 243-260.
2. Maxwell, Hazel, Michelle O'Shea, Megan Stronach, and Sonya Pearce. 2021. "Empowerment through digital health trackers: An exploration of Indigenous Australian women and physical activity in leisure settings." *Annals of Leisure Research* 24:150-167.
3. O'Shea, Michelle, Hazel Maxwell, and Megan Stronach. 2020 "Reconciliatory action and the Gold Coast Commonwealth Games: Inclusion for Indigenous Australian women?" *Sporting Traditions* 37:71-91.
4. O'Shea, Michelle, Hazel Maxwell 2021. "Exploring new media and sport through a gendered lens: enabling possibilities and/or

reproducing inequities for women?". In *Insights on Reporting Sports in the Digital Age: Ethical and Practical Considerations in a Changing Media Landscape*, edited by Roger Domeneghetti: Routledge.

5. O'Shea, Michelle, Hazel Maxwell, Sarah Duffy, and Nicole Peel. 2021. "One step forward and two steps back: pandemic effects and women's sport in Australia". *Restart: Sport After COVID-19. Common Ground.*
6. O'Shea, Michelle, Hazel Maxwell and Sarah Duffy. 2021. "COVID-19 Crisis Response: Did Australian Professional Sport Move Fast Enough". *Time Out: National Perspectives on Sport and the COVID-19 Lockdown. Common Ground.*
7. Richards, Jessica, Michelle O'Shea, Daniela Spanjaard, and Francine Garlin. 2020. 'You can rent it for a while, but it is our house': Sports fans' experience of returning 'home' to a new multipurpose stadium. *International Review for the Sociology of Sport*. Accessed August 25, 2021. doi.org/10.1177/1012690220968570.
8. Stronach, Megan & Michelle O'Shea, M.2021.Learning, understanding and valuing Indigenous peoples' leisure, *Annals of Leisure Research* 24: 1-5.

In: A Closer Look at Women's Health ISBN: 978-1-68507-408-1
Editor: Lakisha Roberts

Chapter 4

EATING DISORDERS IN WOMEN OF COLOR: RACE AND CULTURE-RELATED RISK FACTORS

Shirleen S. Rahman, Sierra A. Thorpe and Regine M. Talleyrand*, PhD
Counseling Program, College of Education and Human Development, George Mason University, Fairfax, VA, USA

ABSTRACT

Lack of research examining Women of Color and eating disorders (EDs) can be attributed to the fact that eating disorders were historically considered to occur only in White women. Yet, current research reports have demonstrated that eating disorder symptoms are a significant problem experienced by *all* women, regardless of race and/or ethnicity. The reported incidences of eating disorder symptoms in Women of Color underscore the need for practitioners to know how to effectively assess and treat *all* individuals who struggle with eating, weight, and body image concerns. Since Women of Color may be less likely to

* Corresponding Author's E-mail: rtalleyr@gmu.edu.

receive referrals or to seek treatment for eating disorder symptoms based partially on prevailing stereotypes of traditional eating disorder clients, cultural mistrust of healthcare systems, fear of stigmatization and/or lack of access to resources, practitioners have an ethical responsibility to provide culturally responsive assessment, prevention and treatment for Women of Color. This chapter will highlight briefly the research that has been conducted among Black/African American, Latinx and Asian American women, review the unique race and culture-related risk factors that may influence the presence of eating disorder symptoms in these populations and provide implications for practitioners.

INTRODUCTION

Lack of research examining Women of Color and eating disorders (EDs) can be attributed to the fact that eating disorders were historically considered to occur only in young, affluent White women (Andersen & Hay, 1985; Root, 2001). Yet, current research reports have demonstrated that eating disorder symptoms are a significant problem experienced by all women, regardless of race and/or ethnicity (Mikhail & Klump, 2020). In fact, African American and Latinx women ED prevalence estimates suggest that Bulimia Nervosa (BN) and Binge Eating Disorder (BED) rates are comparable and/or higher to their White counterparts (Alegria, Woo, Cao, Torres, Meng & Striegel-Moore, 2007; George & Franko, 2010; Rodrigues, 2017) and Asian American women tend to experience similar or higher rates of body dissatisfaction in comparison to their White counterparts (George & Franko, 2010; Grabe & Hyde, 2006; Javier, Moore & Belgrave, 2019).

Researchers have argued that the use of traditional body image measures (i.e., focus on weight and shape) to evaluate appearance satisfaction may obscure the true appearance concerns of Women of Color. Generally speaking, findings from these studies suggest that Women of Color may experience conflicting cultural pressures in the way their beauty and bodies are defined in the dominant culture. Furthermore, Women of Color, as members of two oppressed identity groups (i.e., gender and race) can oftentimes feel objectified, invisible, misunderstood and undervalued when it comes to their bodies and overall appearance (Cheng, Tran, Mikaye, & Kim, 2017; Comas Diaz et al, 2019; Hesse-Biber et al., 2010; Jerald, Cole, Ward, & Avery, 2017). Therefore, fear of additional stigmatization may increase stressors experienced by Women of Color as well as prevent treatment seeking among Women of Color who struggle with eating disorder symptoms and body image concerns (Higgins et al., 2016, Javier & Belgrave, 2019). The purpose of this chapter is to provide a guide for practitioners to better understand how eating disorders and body image are culturally conceptualized among Black/African American, Asian American and Latinx Women. Race and culture specific risk factors such as trauma, acculturation, racism and discrimination, racial/ethnic identity, and comorbidity pathology will be discussed to assist helping professionals in providing culturally responsive practice when working with women of color who struggle with disordered eating and body image concerns.

Women of Color and Eating Disorders

Black/African American Women

Black women are the most studied group of women in the eating disorders literature, with the majority of research studies comparing Black and White women's disordered eating attitudes and behaviors (Grabe & Hyde, 2006, Mikhail & Krump, 2020). Researchers in the past have argued that African American cultural factors may protect against the development of eating disorders in African American women since social pressures surrounding thinness may not exist in the African American community and that African American women, in general, are less likely to view themselves as overweight and less reliant on dieting or weight control behaviors (e.g., Abrams, Allen & Gray, 1993; Javier, Moore & Belgrave, 2016; Smolak & Striegel-Moore, 2001; Thompson, 1994). However, researchers continue to report that prevalence rates of some eating disorder symptoms among African American women are similar to or higher than rates experienced by White women (Shaw, Striegel-Moore, Wilfley, Pike, Dohm, & Fairburn, 2000; Taylor, Caldwell, Baser, Faison, & Jackson, 2007; Mikhai & Klump, 2020). Further, race-related factors (e.g., experiences of racism) may explain who is more susceptible to displaying these symptoms. For example, existing stereotypes (e.g., strong Black woman, hypersexualized Jezebels) used to represent Black women can potentially explain the race-related stressors they may experience (Carter, et al., 2017; Jerald et al., 2017) and the risky eating behaviors (e.g., binge eating) they may use to cope with these stressors (Kempa & Thomas, 2000). On the other hand, African American cultural norms regarding food (e.g., parental pressure ensuring enough food is eaten) can also contribute to maladaptive eating practices in Black children (Lim, Anderson, Hollingsworth, Shepard, Sandridge & Lanciers, 2019). Finally, some researchers claim that Black women do experience pressures regarding beauty and body esteem yet the traditional methods of evaluating these factors (e.g., use of weight, body parts) may not capture the real body appearance concerns of Black Women. That is, additional factors such as hair texture, skin tone, and social comparisons with other Black women may be more relevant when evaluating the body esteem of Black women (Poran, 2006, Talleyrand et al., 2016; Watson, Lewis & Moody, 2019).

Overall, these findings suggest that Black women are not "protected" from experiencing eating disorder symptoms yet may still be misdiagnosed and/or afraid of being stigmatized which can prevent them from seeking treatment. Furthermore, the high rates of obesity and bingeing behaviors in African American women and the inclusion of Binge Eating Disorder (BED) as an official eating disorder in the DSM-V highlight the need to look beyond traditional eating disorders (i.e., anorexia and bulimia) and use of traditional assessments when working with Black/African American women who struggle with problems with eating, weight and shape.

Asian American Women

Asian Americans are the fastest growing racial and ethnic minority group in the United States (Pew Research, 2021), yet have received little attention in eating disorders research (Soh and Walter, 2013, Lee-Winn et al, 2014, Talleyrand, 2013). It has been suggested that this research gap can be related to the stereotypical belief that Asian Americans do not experience psychological problems and their smaller body sizes protect them from experiencing body dissatisfaction (Phan & Tylka, 2006). Others suggest that disordered eating may be under-diagnosed among Asian Americans due to mental health professionals' assumptions that they are well-adjusted (i.e., the "model minority" stereotype; Sue & Suc, 2019). However, research suggests that Asian American women endorse similar and/or higher levels of disordered eating when compared to White women (Franko et al., 2007; Gillen and Lefkowitz, 2012; Akoury, Warren & Culbert, 2019). Some attribute these findings to Asian American women's internalization of sociocultural pressures for thinness from both their traditional and Western cultures (Akoury et al., 2019). Others suggest racially oppressive treatment (e.g., perpetual foreigner hate) or racial objectifications (e.g., depictions of Asian American women as mysterious and hypersexualized) that Asian American women may endure can lead to eating disorder symptoms (Cheng, 2014; Cheng, Tran, Miyake, & Kim, 2017). In addition, Asian Americans potential mistrust of the mental health care system, stigmatized view of mental health disorders, and Asian American cultural values including the need for achievement, perfectionism, and family approval may be reasons why they don't seek help for problems with disordered eating symptoms (Nouri, Hill, & Orrell-Valente, 2011; Phan & Tylka, 2006; Sue & Sue, 2019). Thus, an evaluation of Asian American women's adherence to traditional cultural norms, internalization of sociocultural pressures regarding beauty both within and outside of their traditional cultural standards (i.e., biculturalism), and experiences with racism and discrimination in the US, particularly, gendered racial microaggressions, could be useful when working with Asian American women who present with eating disorder symptoms.

Latinx Women

Latina women represent another rapidly growing majority in the United States yet are also under-represented in the eating disorders research. Some researchers believe that Latina women are protected from being dissatisfied with their bodies since, similar to African American cultural values, curvier body ideals are generally accepted in Latino cultures. Other researchers suggest that adherence to more traditional gender roles and a strong cultural focus on physical appearance may lead to higher prevalence rates of body dissatisfaction among Latina women. In addition, Latino cultural values including the importance of machismo (dominance of men), family, religiosity and simpatia (creating conflict-free situations) may explain why some Latina women may potentially engage in disordered eating behaviors to regulate their emotions (e.g., anger, depression) (Grabe & Hyde, 2006; Talleyrand, 2013; Rodrigues, 2017). A summary of the limited research on Latinx women suggest that they might not engage in dietary restraint behaviors, yet across all other measures of eating disorder symptoms (e.g., weight and shape concerns) rates of eating disorder symptoms are similar to their White female counterparts (Rodrigues, 2017). Thus, whereas some have thought that Latinx women may be protected from internalizing the thin ideal, they still appear to report body and eating behaviors and attitudes characteristic of anorexia, bulimia, and binge-eating disorder which, again, reinforce the fact that cultural factors may no longer "protect" this population.

Another important factor to consider is the rates of obesity in Latinx women since Latinx women have the second highest obesity rates in the United States (US Dept of Health and Human Services, Offices of Minority Health). Some researchers suggest that the acculturation process, a process of adjusting one's own cultural values and belief systems to accommodate the norms and values of a different, more dominate group (Kim & Abreu, 2001), is partially to blame for the obesity problem among Latina immigrants. That is, researchers have found that greater time spent living in the United States after migrating from their indigenous countries has increased the potential for obesity among Latina women and children since they are exposed to new and different dietary patterns and more sedentary lifestyles in the U.S. (Talleyrand, 2013). Thus, an exploration of acculturation stressors and coping strategies, internalization of traditional and dominant cultural norms regarding thinness ideals and overall appearance, and access to food, physical activity and healthcare may be helpful when working with Latinx women who struggle with eating, body image and weight concerns.

Summary

It is evident from increasing literature and prevalence data that Women of Color are displaying rates of eating disorder symptoms similar to or even higher when compared to their White counterparts. Traditional measures used to assess eating disorder symptoms are often based on dominant cultural standards and may not portray an accurate picture of the eating and body appearance concerns Women of Color experience. Thus, a more comprehensive and culturally relevant assessment of eating disorders in Women of Color can assist practitioners with understanding the cultural contexts of these women (Chao et al, 2008; George & Franko, 2010; Goel, Brogan, Boutte, Kaur, & Mazzeo, 2021, Kelly et al., 2011, Rodrigues, 2017). Moreover, increased attention should be given to Asian American and Latina women, since they represent a growing majority of the U.S population and have been marginalized in the eating disorders literature (George & Franko, 2010; Grabe & Hyde, 2006; Warren et al., 2010). Finally, although eating disorder concerns in all women are comparable, White women tend to be more likely to seek out treatment for their eating disorders which further underscores the need for practitioners to increase awareness of ED's, access to ED resources and development of culturally responsive treatment when working with Women of Color.

Race and Culture-Related Risk Factors in Women of Color

We have presented research that dispels the myth that eating disorders only occur in White women and emphasizes how race and cultural factors can influence the manifestation of eating disorder concerns in Women of Color. That is, experiences of racism, discrimination, internalization of indigenous versus dominant culture ideals and acculturative stressors are empirically associated with ED symptoms in Black/African American, Asian American, and Latinx women highlighting these as important variables to include in future research, prevention and clinical treatment when working with these populations (Jerald, Cole, Ward, & Avery, 2017; Mikhail & Klump, 2020).

Racism and Oppression

Researchers have argued that one's experience of differential, unfair treatment based on one's racial group membership can negatively impact both mental health and physical health outcomes (Carter, Lau, Johnson & Kirkinis, 2017; Jerald, Cole, Ward, & Avery, 2017). A related risk factor for the development of eating disorders in Women of Color is their simultaneous membership in two oppressed demographic-identity groups (i.e., gender and race). This membership can heighten the possibility that Women of Color, in particular, will face unique challenges of racism and sexism including feeling marginalized and powerless in society (Jerald et al., 2017; Kempa & Thomas, 2000; Watson et al., 2016). That is, feelings of powerlessness and lack of control, which are common emotions in women who experience eating disorders, could drive Women of Color to use food (e.g., either restricting food or bingeing) as a mechanism to gain back control in their lives (Kempa & Thomas, 2000, Thompson, 1994, Talleyrand, 2013, Talleyrand, 2016). Given that Women of Color's eating and health concerns may be related to the double jeopardy of being a Person of Color and female, it is imperative that practitioners are aware of the interaction of racism and sexism and how it may contribute to eating disorder symptoms in Women of Color. Practitioners should also assess perceived stereotypes among Women of Color who present with ED symptoms based on the fact that perceived discrimination and gendered racial microaggressions may increase the risk for ED symptoms in People of Color (Kelly, 2018).

Acculturative Stressors

Acculturation has often been viewed as the phenomenon that occurs when an individual comes into contact with more than one cultural system (Padilla, 1980). Thus, the acculturation process entails adjusting one's cultural values and belief systems to accommodate the norms and values of a different, more dominant group. Conversely, enculturation is a process through which an individual retains his or her own cultural values regardless of the dominant culture (Kim & Abreu, 2001). For example, a female immigrant from El Salvador living in the United States can be considered acculturated if she adopts the "sociocultural pursuit of thinness" embedded in the U.S. dominant culture but enculturated if she retains the cultural norms defining beauty and appearance from her country of origin (Talleyrand, 2013). Acculturative stressors include trying to assimilate to the majority culture's beauty standards, values and practices, and is associated with general psychological distress as well as negative physical health issues (Kroon Van Diest et al., 2014). The perceived beauty standard portrayed within Western society has traditionally been Eurocentric features like White skin, thin frame, small nose, and lighter hair and eyes. This standard of beauty is often unrealistic for Women of Color and attempts to attain a thin body frame can result in eating disorder symptoms and internalized resentment (Kroon Van Diest et al., 2014).

A study conducted by Perez at al., (2002), found acculturative stress to be a contributor to eating disorder behaviors, such as bulimic symptoms, among a group of Latina and African American women (Kroon Van Diest et al., 2014). This study by Perez et al., (2002), indicated that women of these ethnic backgrounds who had higher levels of acculturative stress and body dissatisfaction showed symptoms of bulimia. In comparison, women who were also in these ethnic groups who did not suffer from acculturative stress, did not show symptoms of bulimia, even if they were dissatisfied with their bodies (Kroon Van Diest et al., 2014). These results emphasis the importance of evaluating how Women of Color are internalizing dominant cultural standards of beauty.

Another way acculturative stress can affect Women of Color and eating pathology is from events that have happened historically to their racial and/or ethnic group (Ross et al., 2018). Specifically, but not limited to African American and Native American women, negative historical events can exacerbate acculturative stress, which can lead to things like binge eating disorder as a maladaptive way of coping (Ross et al., 2018). As cited in Ross et al., (2018), a study conducted by Clark and Winterowd (2012), revealed that acts of systemic oppression like slavery, racism, forced assimilation, and discrimination are all factors that contribute to binge eating disorder in African American Women. Similarly, another study conducted by Clark and Winterowd (2012) found the stress of historical oppression on a group of Native American women may have influenced their eating pathology, leading to binge eating disorder (Ross et al., 2018). Asian American women have additional pressures from their own culture and have to navigate traditional Asian values and Westernized culture, making it difficult when developing their racial identity (Obleada & Bennett, 2021). These findings show the strong links between experiences of racism, oppression and acculturation stressors and the manifestation of ED symptoms in Women of Color.

Racial and Ethnic Identity

The concept of racial identity is related to the extent to which the person identifies with the racial group to which he or she supposedly belongs with the belief that commitment to one's racial group is necessary for healthy psychological functioning (Helms & Cook, 1999). Ethnic identity refers to the extent women accept, identify with and affirm their ethnic heritage (Phinney, 1992). Researchers have suggested that high levels of ethnic and racial identity may assist ethnically diverse women in rejecting the societal beauty ideals of the dominant culture (Harris, 1994; Shuttlesworth & Zotter, 2011; Wood & Petrie, 2010; Williams et al., 2019). However, Women of Color who idealize dominant cultural ideals often experience body dissatisfaction, and tend to struggle with their racial identity and/or ethnic identity (Flowers et al., 2011). According to Flowers et al., (2011), African American women who have not entirely affirmed their racial and ethnic heritage are more vulnerable to adopting and internalizing the Western society's thin ideal. This, in turn, may cause maladaptive eating behaviors and high levels of body dissatisfaction. In comparison, African American women who identify their Blackness as a salient part of their identity, usually report less psychological turmoil and a higher self-esteem (Javier et al, 2016; Flowers et al., 2011). It appears that, for African American women, a strong racial identity can serve as a protective factor against internalized Eurocentric beauty standards and eating pathology (Obleada & Bennett, 2021).

As for Asian American women, a strong ethnic identity may actually lead to experiencing eating disorder symptoms since many Asian cultures tend to idealize thinness when compared to other cultures of color. This could increase Asian American women's risks of experiencing body dissatisfaction and disordered eating patterns (Obleada & Bennett, 2021).

In fact, studies have found that Asian American women who strongly identified with traditional Asian values had a higher level of body dissatisfaction (Lau et al., 2006; Obleada & Bennett, 2021). These findings suggest that depending on the racial and/or ethnic group, a strong racial or ethnic identity can serve as a protective or risk factor when it comes to susceptibility to experiencing eating disorders.

TRAUMA

Trauma has a variety of definitions in mental healthcare and its influence on other mental health disorders is crucial but often overlooked. Trauma and symptoms associated with trauma disorders (i.e., Post-Traumatic Stress Disorder (PTSD) are often present in those diagnosed with eating disorders. Several studies identified the connection between traumatic events, PTSD symptoms, and eating disorder diagnoses (Brewerton, 2007; Groth et al., 2019; Holzer et al., 2008; Rienecke et al., 2020). Traumatic events that include violence, abuse, and neglect are typically discussed in the existing literature on the relationship with trauma and eating disorders. However, the interaction of culture and trauma are important to consider as there are various ways trauma can manifest in eating disorders because of cultural impacts. One study on Black women, binge eating, and trauma discussed how the internalization of a "Strong Black Woman" influenced emotional regulation in relation to binge eating and processing traumatic events (Harrington et al., 2010). Specifically, this study identified a key cultural phenomenon specific to Black women that influenced the etiology of an eating disorder in addition to the impact of trauma.

As previously stated, culture is crucial when exploring trauma and other risk factors for eating disorders and ignoring cultural influences can cause key risk factors to be ignored by practitioners working with eating disorders. Specifically, racialized trauma is a form of trauma that is not always recognized during an initial assessment for trauma history.

However, it is crucial to acknowledge how various forms of racism, discrimination, and prejudice can affect the person's overall mental well-being. One study connected how racial and sexual objectification of Asian women led to higher rates of trauma symptomology and disordered eating (Cheng & Youngju Kim, 2018). Additionally, this article emphasized that long term oppression from racism and sexism is complex and multi-layered but crucial when exploring risk factors and etiology of body image issues and disordered eating habits (Cheng & Youngju Kim, 2018).

Additionally, sexual trauma and abuse appear to be common when assessing trauma history for individuals with various eating disorders (Brewerton. 2007; Groth et al., 2019; Holzer et al., 2008). A study on adolescents with eating disorders reported that assessing for trauma history is a critical piece of eating disorder treatment since there is overlap between the lack of control when it comes to both trauma and eating disorder symptoms (Groth et al., 2019). Another study linked higher rates of childhood sexual abuse history with bulimia compared to all other eating disorders (Brewerton, 2007). Trauma can cause a person to feel out of control with their life in a variety of ways and disorders can manifest as a way of obtaining that control. Eating disorders often involve a level of control that parallels an addiction to drugs or alcohol where there is constant fixation. This sense of control can often placate the pain that is rooted deeper from traumatic events.

Also, Women of Color disproportionately experience trauma at a more complex level as it relates to various forms of oppression such as racism and sexual objectification (Watson et al., 2016). Thus, it is important to have an intersectional based approach when assessing and treating women of color regardless of the presenting mental health issues because trauma can cut across generations, individual events, and systemic factors (Watson et al., 2016). Overall, trauma is a significant and multi-layered risk factor for eating disorders and disordered eating behavior. This portion alluded to comorbidity of other mental health disorders with eating disorders, but a more in-depth analysis of comorbidity with eating disorders is explored in the next section.

Comorbid Pathology

Mental Health Comorbidity

As previously mentioned, eating disorders affect many aspects of a person's life, and often times can lead to the onset of another mental illness. Eating disorders pose specific issues for patients, and tend to continue over an extended period of time, giving unintentional space for the comorbidity of other disorders to form (Martín et al., 2019). Relatedly, individuals who develop eating disorders can also have a pre-existing mental health diagnosis. Studies have shown that the development of an anxiety disorder often times proceeds developing an eating disorder, leading some researchers to believe anxiety is a potential medical pathway to an ED (Swinebourne et al., 2012). Comorbidity may complicate the diagnostic and treatment process with patients who suffer from eating disorders (Martín et al., 2019). This may be because the mental illness could be a risk factor for the eating disorder, or could be secondary to the eating disorder (Swinebourne et al., 2012). Blinder et al., (2006) report that around 67% of women in-patients with eating disorders have an anxiety disorder, and around 90% have depression (Martín et al., 2019). A multitude of studies have shown that major depressive disorder is the most prevalent comorbid mental illness in ED patients (Martín et al., 2019). Given that race and culture related stressors may cause detrimental mental health effects (e.g., depression) in Women of Color (Carter et al., 2017), it is important to assess for co-existing mental health concerns when working with Women of Color who present with ED symptoms.

Medical Comorbidity

Eating disorders are classified as a mental illness, but this is also a disease of the body and often causes severe, and sometimes irreversible damage. Some of the possible effects are malnutrition, infertility, loss of teeth enamel, physical health issues, stress fractures, obesity, cardiac arrest, and even death (Kroon Van Diest et al., 2014). Medical professionals should be screening for eating disorders, but not only when someone is noticeably underweight or obese. Women of Color may struggle with eating disorders that may not be readily apparent yet traditional assumptions regarding how eating disorder patients should "look" (i.e., identify as White) can lead to misdiagnosis in Women of Color. Furthermore, when it comes to Women of Color, additional race and culture-related stressors may contribute to the development of an eating disorder, as well as the development of other medical issues (Ross et al., 2018). African American women are at an exceedingly high risk of developing obesity, and binge eating disorder (BED) is most prevalent among this population as well (Ross et al., 2018). Comorbidity of BED and obesity is something that medical professionals should be assessing for when it comes to this population (Jaiswal, 2019).

IMPLICATIONS FOR PRACTITIONERS

We have discussed race and culture-related stressors that may be correlated with the prevalence of eating disorder and body image concerns in Black/African American, Asian American, and Latinx women. Given the increasing diversity in the United States, practitioners should be aware of varied cultural norms within each group as well as race and culture correlates that that go beyond personal variables (e.g., perfectionism, anxiety) when assessing disordered eating and body image concerns in Women of Color. In addition, trauma and comorbidity factors may be linked to racial and cultural norms and experiences so it is important to consider these factors when assessing ED's in Women of Color. Relatedly, from a historical perspective, Women of Color may experience medical distrust based on previous misdiagnoses (Jaiswal, 2019), so it is imperative that practitioners create safe and trusting spaces for Women of Color. Finally, practitioners should be aware that each racial and/or ethnic group is not monolithic and that examining intersecting identities (e.g., levels of acculturation, racial identity, cultural norms based on geographical location) within their patient/client populations are warranted (Jerald et al., 2017).

Increased Awareness of and Advocacy for Diverse Cultural Norms

Our findings suggest that utilizing a contextual and intersectional framework when examining the experiences of Women of Color is imperative; otherwise, researchers and practitioners may overlook risk and protective factors that are unique to these populations.

Practitioners should be particularly cognizant of how traditional cultural norms, stereotyping, stigmatization, misdiagnosis, and lack of ED education and access to healthcare may compromise Women of Color's mental and physical health. Understanding how a client's level of acculturation to her traditional culture or the dominant culture influences her beliefs regarding food and physical appearance is critical. Therefore, assessing levels of acculturation and enculturation with clients can provide useful information on how and why clients present with weight concerns. Potential questions to pose with clients who have experienced the acculturation process could include migration status, generational status, rationale for coming to the United States, language acquisition, duration of time spent in the United States, lack of family presence and race and/or ethnicity of social networks (Talleyrand, 2013). Also examining lack of privilege (s) (e.g., race, class, citizenship) among patients/clients can assist practitioners with understanding additional contextual stressors that may exist on top of normal life stressors. Furthermore, we suggest that helping professionals engage in mandatory trainings related to increasing awareness regarding diverse cultural group norms, understanding experiences of acculturation and enculturation and experiences of racism and oppression so that those who may be at risk (intentionally or unintentionally) of perpetrating microaggressions, cultural mistrust and misdiagnoses in their practice may be prevented from doing so.

Use of Culturally Relevant Assessments

Eating disorders are often mystified in healthcare and are seen as a population of individuals with acute needs and high-risk factors. However, factors that contribute to disordered eating behavior and eating disorders exist in daily life for everyone. Women experience a bombardment of messages related to food, their bodies, and diet culture from a young age and can internalize these as they grow up. Later, these messages can manifest into a myriad of issues related to weight, food, and body image. Upon formal diagnoses, an eating disorder can be an extremely stigmatized mental health condition, and the conversations around it focus heavily on treatment rather than prevention or etiology of the disorder. Assessments are a crucial piece to understanding how eating disorders and disordered eating behaviors manifest. Additionally, assessments can provide a variety of professionals an opportunity to engage in prevention and early interventions as opposed to a higher level of care that is stereotypically associated with eating disorders (e.g., Rodriguez et al., 2008).

A study examining trends on assessments for eating disorders found that how self-report measures and the use of formal assessments with high validity have significantly increased in the past decade (Towne et al., 2017). Additionally, it was found that unstructured interviews alone were not sufficient measures for assessing an eating disorder (Towne et al., 2017). This further emphasizes the role that assessment plays in both treating and preventing eating disorders. Assessing for eating disorders should not be exclusively clinical or symptom-based, especially if prevention is a focus. Often, people will deny having an eating disorder or disordered eating behavior simply because of how the question is phrased to avoid stigma or other negative reactions.

Lastly, assessments must be culturally relevant and tailored for the person or population being assessed. If an assessment is not culturally competent or offers flexibility to adapt to different cultural norms beyond dominant idealized standards of beauty, then it may not be as effective and engaging for the person receiving it. For example, when evaluating eating disorder symptoms and appearance in Women of Color, it can also be useful to assess areas that go beyond weight and shape (i.e., facial features, skin tone, hair texture) since these have been found to be equally important appearance factors in Women of Color (Goel et al., 2021; Talleyrand et al., 2016; Watson et al., 2019). Practitioners conducting ED assessments should also endorse creating a safe, egalitarian and collaborative environment to reduce any stigma regarding eating disorders since Women of Color may be experiencing some sense of shame and/or lack of information regarding eating disorders and their related symptoms. Some potential questions to use are included below:

- How were you raised to understand food, body image and overall appearance in your life?
- How would you describe your current relationship with food? With your body?
- What are your current eating habits like?
- What is your typical eating pattern/routine?
- How much do you want weight incorporated into your health goals?
- Are there any meals that you skip or omit?
- Do you wish to change anything about your relationship with food?
- What influences your relationship with your body?
- Are there are current life changes impacting your eating habits? Feelings towards your body image? Overall appearance?
- Have you noticed any significant changes in weight? *
- *Significant weight gain AND weight loss can indicate disordered eating

In addition, use of the RESPECTFUL model (D'Andrea & Daniels, 2001) can provide practitioners with a more contextual framework for understanding the lived experiences of the individuals they are working with. The letters in the RESPECTFUL acronym represent the following topics to explore: religious identity, economic background, sexual and/or gender identity, personal style/education, ethnic/racial identity, chronological lifespan, trauma, family background, and location/language (D'Andrea & Daniels 2001). Use of this model is emphasized in the case studies provided below.

CASE STUDIES

Case Study 1

Shannon is a 28-year-old African American bisexual female who arrives to outpatient therapy to treat her binge eating disorder. She arrives for her initial intake and reports that she struggled with binge eating disorder since she finished college. It was gathered from the intake that she grew up receiving mixed messages about her body type from her family and was sexually assaulted at a college party during her junior year of college. Currently, she is struggling with intimate relationships and reported that rejection is a significant trigger for her bingeing.

Case Study 1 Suggestions

- Utilize the RESPECTFUL counseling framework to explore client's intersecting identities (e.g., race, sexuality, age, gender, racial and ethnic identity). This model should be used once a safe counseling environment is established through rapport building and open discussion.
- Explore how/if her sexual trauma impacted her during college

- Consider family dynamics and how it impacted her body image and eating behaviors (e.g., mixed messages growing up; parental endorsement of eating behaviors)
- Validating the reason behind the client's binge eating while simultaneously working on behavioral changes to address binging
- Exploring her identified trigger and consider possible connection to her sexual trauma, which could impact intimacy as well.

Case Study 2

Noora is a 35-year-old straight married Indian American female who arrives to outpatient therapy after recently relapsing with her bulimia. She has approximately five years in recovery from her bulimia, but reported she recently relapsed after living with her in-laws for approximately 6 months prior who immigrated from India. She reported that her culture was triggering at times but felt that she could manage it since she has spent several years in recovery but is looking to begin therapy again as she works on recovery.

Case Study 2 Suggestions

- Utilize the RESPECTFUL counseling framework to explore client's intersecting identities (i.e., race, sexuality, age, gender, etc.). This model should be used once a safe counseling environment is established through rapport building and open discussion.
- Explore the connection between family and cultural values in Asian cultures
- Explore how body image, weight, and food are discussed currently
- Re-establish and reinforce existing behaviors that existed while client was in recovery

- Connect client with proper nutritional rehabilitation providers if necessary
- Examine how client was able to maintain recovery and build on existing strengths

CONCLUSION

Research has shown that Women of Color do experience disordered eating and body image concerns at rates that are often comparable to their White counterparts. Furthermore, race and culture do impact eating pathology therefore practitioners need to consider cultural conceptualizations of ED's and body image when working with Women of Color. Many Women of Color may face many barriers to receiving care for EDs, including limited understanding of and availability of care, cultural mistrust of healthcare systems, stigma within their communities, and potential stereotyping, misdiagnosis and lack of culturally competent assessment from practitioners. Further, there are unique within group differences (e.g., subsets of Asian Americans) in factors that could affect eating pathology within racial/ethnic groups therefore practitioners should not assume that all members of a racial and/or ethnic group is the same. While this chapter presents meaningful ways to contribute to our understanding of EDs and body image concerns in Black/African American, Asian American, and Latinx Women, we need to continue to increase representation of their lived experiences through research (both qualitative and quantitative) and also strive to develop culturally relevant assessment, prevention and treatment practices. We also need to explore experiences of Arab American and Native American women since research in this area is virtually nonexistent. Finally, we should increase our understanding of bi-racial identity populations since this is the fastest growing racial group in the US and also a group that has been underrepresented in the eating disorders literature.

References

Akoury, L. M., Warren, C. S., & Culbert, K. M. (2019). Disordered Eating in Asian American Women: Sociocultural and Culture Specific Factors. *Frontiers in Psychology, 10,* 1-11.

Andersen, A. E., & Hay, A. (1985). Racial and socioeconomic influences in anorexia and bulimia. *International Journal of Eating Disorders, 4,* 479-487.

Berry, J. W. (1998). Acculturative stress. *Handbook of Multicultural Perspectives on Stress and Coping*, 287–298. https://doi.org/10.1007/0-387-26238-5_12.

Carter, R. T., Lau, M. Y., Johnson, V., & Kirkinis, K. (2017). Racial Discrimination and Health Outcomes Among Racial/Ethnic Minorities: A Meta-Analytic Review. *Journal of Multicultural Counseling and Development, 45,* 232-259.

Chao, Y. M., Pisetsky, B. A., Dierker, L. C., Dohm, F., Rosselli, F., May A. M., & Striegel-Moore, R.H. (2008). Ethnic differences in weight control practices among U.S. adolescents from 1995-2005. *International Journal of Eating Disorders, 41: 2,* 124-133.

Cheng, H. L. (2014). Disordered eating among Asian/Asian American women: Racial and cultural factors as correlates. *The Counseling Psychologist, 42(6),* 821–851. https://doi-org.proxy-um.researchport.umd.edu/10.1177/0011000014535472.

Cheng, H. L., Tran, A. G., Miyake, E. R., & Kim, H. Y. (2017). Disordered eating among Asian American college women: A racially expanded model of objectification theory. *Journal of Counseling Psychology, 64(2),* 179–191. https://doi-org.proxy-um.researchport.umdedu/10. 1037/cou0000195.

Brewerton, T. D. (2007). Eating disorders, trauma, and comorbidity: Focus on PTSD. E*ating Disorders, 15*(4), 285–304. https://doi.org/10. 1080/10640260701454311.

D'Andrea, M., & Daniels, J. (2001). RESPECTFUL counseling: An integrative model for counselors. In D. Pope-Davis & H. Coleman

(Eds.), *The interface of class, culture and gender in counseling* (pp.417-466). Thousand Oaks, CA: Sage.

Flowers, K. C., Levesque, M. J., & Fischer, S. (2011). The relationship between maladaptive eating behaviors and racial identity Among African American women in college. *Journal of Black Psychology, 38*(3), 290–312. https://doi.org/10.1177/0095798411416459.

Gerbasi, M. E., Richards, L. K., Thomas, J. J., Agnew-Blais, J. C., Thompson-Brenner, H., Gilman, S. E., & Becker, A. E. (2014). Globalization and eating disorder risk: Peer influence, perceived social norms, and adolescent disordered eating in Fiji. *International Journal of Eating Disorders, 47(7)*, 727–737.

Goel, N. J., Brogan, T, Boutte, R. L., Kaur, B., & Mazzeo, S.E. (2021). Body Image and Eating Disorders Among South Asian American Women: What Are We Missing? *Qualitative Health Research,* 1-16. https://doi.org/10.1177/10497323211036896.

Goode, R. W., Cowell, M. M., Mazzeo, S. E., Cooper-Lewter, C., Forte, A., Olayia, O. I., & Bulik, C. M. (2020). Binge eating and binge-eating disorder in black women: A systematic review. *International Journal of Eating Disorders, 53(4),* 491–507.

Grabe, S., & Hyde, J.S. (2006). Ethnicity and body dissatisfaction among women in the United States: A meta-analysis. *Psychological Bulletin, 132,* 622-640.

Groth, T., Hilsenroth, M., Boccio, D., & Gold, J. (2019). Relationship between trauma history and eating disorders in adolescents. *Journal of Child & Adolescent Trauma, 13*(4), 443–453. https://doi.org/ 10.1007/ s40653-019-00275-z.

Harrington, E. F., Crowther, J. H., & Shipherd, J. C. (2010). Trauma, binge eating, and the "strong Black woman." *Journal of Consulting and Clinical Psychology, 78*(4), 469–479. https://doi.org/10.1037/ a0019174.

Helms, J. E. & Cook, D. A. (1999). *Using race and culture in counseling and psychotherapy: Theory and process*. Upper Saddle River, NJ: Pearson, Allyn, and Bacon.

Holzer, S. R., Uppala, S., Wonderlich, S. A., Crosby, R. D., & Simonich, H. (2008). Mediational significance of PTSD in the relationship of sexual trauma and eating disorders. *Child Abuse & Neglect, 32*(5), 561–566. https://doi.org/10.1016/j.chiabu.2007.07.011.

Jaiswal, J. (2019). Whose responsibility is it to dismantle medical mistrust? Future directions for researchers and health care providers. *Behavioral Medicine*, *45*(2), 188–196. https://doi.org/10.1080/08964289.2019. 1630357.

Javier, S. J., Moore, M. P., Belgrave, F. Z. (2016). Racial comparisons in perception of maternal and peer attitudes, body dissatisfaction, and eating disorders among African American and White women. *Women & Health, 56,* 615– 633.

Kempa, M. L., & Thomas, A. J. (2000). Culturally sensitive assessment and treatment of eating disorders. *Eating Disorders, 8:1,* 7-12. doi: 1064-0266/00.

Kim, B. S. K., & Abreu, J. M. (2001). Acculturation measurement: Theory, current instruments, and future directions. In J. G. Ponterotto, J. M. Casas, L. A. Suzuki, & C. M. Alexander (Eds.), *Handbook of multicultural counseling* (2nd ed., pp. 394–424). Thousand Oaks, CA: Sage.

Le, T., Kuo, L, & Yamasaki, V. (2020). Gendered Racial Microaggressions, Feminism, and Asian American Women's Eating Pathology: An Intersectional Approach. *Sex Roles, 83, 127-142.* https://doi.org/10.1007/s11199-019-01100-5.

Lim, C. S., Anderson, L. M., Hollingsworth, D. W., Shepherd, L., Sandridge, S. & Lanciers, S. (2019). Comparing disordered eating and feeding practices in African American and Caucasian treatment-seeking youth with obesity. *Eating Disorders, 27, 2,* 152-167. https://doi.org/10.1080/10640266.2019.1614825.

Martín, J., Arostegui, I., Loroño, A., Padierna, A., Najera-Zuloaga, J., & Quintana, J. M. (2019). Anxiety and depressive symptoms are related to core symptoms, general health outcome, and medical comorbidities in eating disorders. *European Eating Disorders Review*, *27*(6), 603–613. https://doi.org/10.1002/erv.2677.

Mikhail, M & Klump, K. (2020). A virtual issue highlighting eating disorders in people of Black/African and Indigenous heritage. *International Journal of Eating Disorders,* 459-466, DOI: 10.1002/eat.23402.

Mitchell, J. E. (2015). Medical comorbidity and medical complications associated with binge-eating disorder. *International Journal of Eating Disorders*, *49*(3), 319–323. https://doi.org/10.1002/eat.22452.

Navarro-Haro, M. V., Botella, C., Guillen, V., Moliner, R., Marco, H., Jorquera, M., Baños, R., & Garcia-Palacios, A. (2018). Dialectical behavior therapy in the treatment of borderline personality disorder and eating disorders comorbidity: A pilot study in a naturalistic setting. *Cognitive Therapy and Research*, *42*(5), 636–649. https://doi.org/10. 1007/s10608-018-9906-9.

Nicdao, E. G., Hong, S., Takeuchi, D. T. (2007). Prevalence and correlates of eating disorders among Asian Americans: Results from the National Latino and Asian American Study. *International Journal of Eating Disorders, 40,* S22-S26.

Obleada, K. T., & Bennett, B. L. (2021). Moderation effects of Ethnic-Racial identity on Disordered eating and Ethnicity among Asian and Caucasian Americans. *Frontiers in Psychology*, *12*. https://doi.org/ 10.3389/fpsyg.2021.594391.

Padilla, A. (Ed.). (1980). *Acculturation: Theory, models, and some new findings*. Boulder, CO: Westview.

Phan, T., & Tylka, T. C. (2006). Exploring a model and moderators of disordered eating with Asian American college women. *Journal of Counseling Psychology, 53 (1),* 36-47.

Rienecke, R. D., Blalock, D. V., Duffy, A., Manwaring, J., Le Grange, D., Johnson, C., Mehler, P. S., & McClanahan, S. F. (2021). Posttraumatic stress disorder symptoms and trauma-informed care in higher levels of care for eating disorders. *The International Journal of Eating Disorders,* *54*(4), 627–632. https://doi.org/ 10.1002/eat.23455.

Rodrigues, M (2017). Do Hispanic Girls Develop Eating Disorders? A Critical Review of the Literature. *Hispanic Health Care International, 15, 4,* 189-196.

Root, M. P. P. (2001). Future considerations in research on eating disorders. *The Counseling Psychologist, 29,* 754-762.

Shaw, H., Ramirez, L., Trost, A., Randall, P., & Stice, E. (2004). Body image and eating disturbances across ethnic groups: More similarities than differences. *Psychology of Addictive Behaviors, 18*, 12-18.

Smolak, L., & Striegel-Moore, R. H. (2001). Challenging the myth of the golden girl: Ethnicity and eating disorders. In R. H. Striegel-Moore and L. Smolak (Eds.), *Eating disorders: Innovative directions in research and practice* (pp. 111-132). American Psychological Association: Washington, DC.

Sue, D.W & Sue, D (2019). *Counseling the culturally diverse: Theory and practice (8th ed.).* Hoboken: John Wiley & Sons, Inc.

Swinbourne, J., Hunt, C., Abbott, M., Russell, J., St Clare, T., & Touyz, S. (2012). The comorbidity between eating disorders and anxiety disorders: Prevalence in an eating disorder sample and anxiety disorder sample. *Australian & New Zealand Journal of Psychiatry, 46*(2), 118–131. https://doi.org/10.1177/0004867411432071.

Talleyrand, R.M. (2013). Clients of Color and Eating Disorders: Cultural Considerations. In *Eating Disorders and Obesity: A Counselor's Guide to Treatment and Prevention*. American Counseling Association Press.

Talleyrand, R.M., Gordon, A, D., Daquin, J.V., & Johnson, A.J. (2016). Expanding our understanding of eating attitudes, eating practices and body image in African American Women: A qualitative study. *Journal of Black Psychology*, 1-29, doi: 10.1177/0095798416649086.

Taylor, J. Y., Caldwell, C. H., Baser, R. E., Faison, N., & Jackson, J. S. (2007). Prevalence of eating disorders among Blacks in the National Survey of American Life. *International Journal of Eating Disorders, 40,* S10-S14.

Thompson, B. (1994). *A hunger so wide and so deep.* Minneapolis, MN: University of Minnesota Press.

Thompson, B. (1997). Multiracial feminist theorizing about eating: Refusing to rank oppressions. *Eating Disorders: The Journal of Treatment & Prevention, 4*, 104-114.

Towne, T. L., De Young, K. P., & Anderson, D. A. (2017). Trends in professionals' use of eating disorder assessment instruments. *Professional Psychology, Research and Practice, 48*(4), 243–250. https://doi.org/10.1037/pro0000067.

Watson, L. B., DeBlaere, C., Langrehr, K. J., Zelaya, D. G., & Flores, M. J. (2016). The influence of multiple oppressions on women of color's experiences with insidious trauma. *Journal of Counseling Psychology, 63*(6), 656–667. https://doi.org/10.1037/cou0000165.

Watson, L. B, Lcwis, J. A., & Moody, A. T. (2019). A sociocultural examination of body image among Black Women. *Body Image, 31,* 280-287.

Biographical Sketches

Regine Mylene Talleyrand

Affiliation: George Mason University, Counseling Program

Education: PhD in Counseling Psychology

Research and Professional Experience: Dr. Regine Talleyrand is an Associate Professor for the Counseling Program in the College of Education and Human Development at George Mason University. She completed her PhD in Counseling Psychology from the University of Maryland and received her Bachelor of Arts degree in Psychology from the University of Pennsylvania. Dr. Talleyrand has spent the past twenty years studying mental and physical health disparities in People of Color and developing culturally relevant counseling interventions for communities that have been underrepresented and underserved. She has published and presented extensively in the areas of eating disorders in

People of Color, racial and ethnic identity development, acculturation stressors for immigrant populations, multicultural social justice counseling, career counseling and advising and mentoring relationships.

Professional Appointments: George Mason University, College of Education and Human Development, Counseling Program: Assistant Professor (2001-2007); Associate Professor, 2007-present.

Publications from the Last 3 Years:

Chung, R. C-Y., Bemak, F., Talleyrand, R. M. & Williams, J. (2018). Challenges in promoting race dialogues in psychology training: Race and gender perspectives. *The Counseling Psychologist, 46, 2,* 213-240, doi-org.mutex.gmu.edu/10. 1177/001100 0018758262.

Stewardson, L., Nolan, J.R., & Talleyrand, R. M. (2020). Eating Disorders and Body Image Concerns in Men of Color: Cultural Considerations. *Journal of Mental Health Counseling,* 42 (2): 110–123. https://doi.org/10.17744/mehc.42.2.02.

Talleyrand, R. M., & Vojtech, J. (2018). Potential stressors of undocumented Latinx youth: Implications and recommendations for school counselors. *Professional School Counseling, 22*(1). https://doi.org/10.1177/2156759X19847168.

Shirleen Shanta Rahman

Affiliation: George Mason University, Counseling Program

Education: BS in Psychology

Research and Professional Experience: Shirleen Rahman is currently a master's-level graduate student at George Mason University's Counseling and Development Program. Her concentration is in Clinical Mental Health Counseling. She completed her bachelor's degree in

Psychology at Virginia Tech in 2017. Throughout her undergraduate career, she worked in a research lab that focused on behavioral science and conducted research on a variety of topics ranging from healthy habits to safety behaviors. She co-authored various presentations and presented at a conference on applied behavioral analysis as well. After entering her graduate program in 2019, she began working for the local community services board at an in-patient facility for people with substance use disorders. Currently she is finishing up her final semester in her master's program and interning at a countywide organization that serves survivors of domestic violence, sexual violence, human trafficking, and stalking. Throughout her experience in the counseling program, her interests began to focus on mental health concerns for People of Color in community settings, survivors of domestic and sexual violence, and co-occurring issues with substance use and trauma disorders. Her current research interests focus on South Asian populations in mental health disorders and traumatic experiences.

Sierra Ashley Thorpe

Affiliation: George Mason University, Counseling Program

Education: BS in Psychology

Research and Professional Experience: Sierra Thorpe is currently in her third year of her Master's program studying Clinical Mental Health Counseling at George Mason University. She completed her bachelor's degree in Psychology at Old Dominion University in 2017. Throughout her undergraduate career, she served as Kappa Delta's Vice President of community service, and facilitated self-esteem and mentoring workshops with Girl Scouts of the USA. She also completed a psychology practicum as an intern at an elementary school for children with behavioral disorders. After beginning her graduate program in January of 2019, she worked at a rehabilitation facility for drugs and alcohol as a program assistant. She also worked at a group home for at risk youth as a residential counselor. Currently, she interns at a non-profit, known as The Women's Center, providing therapy to people of all ages who struggle with things like anxiety, depression, eating disorders, trauma, grief and loss, and PTSD. Her current interests center around children and adolescents, co-occurring issues surrounding grief and trauma, and women of color and their unique struggles. As for research, she is particularly drawn to the possible connection of racial identity development and eating disorders in women of color.

In: A Closer Look at Women's Health
Editor: Lakisha Roberts
ISBN: 978-1-68507-408-1

Chapter 5

The Body Asks and the Mind Judges: Understanding Desires and Food Cravings in Eating Behavior and Its Triggers

Jônatas de Oliveira*
Eating Disorders Program (AMBULIM/PROTAD),
Institute of Psychiatry, University of Sao Paulo, Sao Paulo, Brazil
School of Medicine, University of Sao Paulo, Sao Paulo, Brazil

Abstract

One of the aspects involved in the motivation for food consumption and the physiological need for food is Desires for food and Food Cravings. Although there are several definitions for Food Craving in the literature, it is currently understood as a cognitive event involving emotional, physiological, and external aspects. Desires, when intense, also involve torture and awareness of a lack (i.e., Food Craving) which is associated with the diet mentality and cognitive restraint and also

* Corresponding Author's E-mail: oliveira.jonatas@usp.br.

associations between affectivity, environment present in Disordered Eating and Eating Disorders cases, which suffer from the greater intensity of Food Craving compared to individuals without Eating Disorders. In this chapter, I deal with the history and definition of Food Craving, the description of the cognitive event of appetizing targeting, the associations with the diet mentality as a promoter of moral judgment concerning food, and the twelve primary triggers (external: positive/negative events, food environment, advertising, cultural beliefs about food, specific places, the food itself and internal triggers: dietary restraint, food reward, impulsivity/inflexibility, emotions/thoughts/ feelings about food, hunger/satiety/appetite and finally, anxiety and depression symptoms) according to the latest data from studies in the field of Eating Disorders. Finally, it is the nutritional treatment of Food Cravings in cases of Disordered Eating and Eating Disorders that involve cognitive approaches aimed at eating behavior and the involvement of the principles of Intuitive Eating and the satisfaction of food desires and FC's treatment.

Keywords: food craving, eating disorders, binge eating disorder, bulimia nervosa, anorexia nervosa

1. INTRODUCTION

1.1. Definition and Historic

Defining Food Craving (FC) is a research challenge that has proved to be controversial in the literature many times. First, we will define the concept of desire, as craving represents a dimension that involves the recruitment of some mechanisms of intensification and attentional focus. The most mentioned article on the subject in the literature presents the term phenomenology, being entitled "The phenomenology of food cravings," published in 1990 by Weingarten and Elston. The theoretical construction within this text does not have a phrase that defines FC, due to the complexity of the theme [1]. The following year, the same authors created a questionnaire to analyze FC, with clear efforts to measure and categorize the construct. As it is a hypothetical construction, desire suffers from several problems related to its definition, because it is not directly measurable or observable.

Just before Weingarten and Elston's publication, some researchers postulated that "desire functions as a method of protection against anguish, alerting the individual to a potential source of relief" [2, 3], but it was not until 1987 that an important debate was carried out about the concept, when two researchers published an article mentioning the various uses of craving in research on the use of different substances. In this text, they suggest craving as "strong desire or intense longing," asking researchers to be cautious in the use of craving, as a terminology of more cultural jargon [4]. Several analyzes on the use of craving were presented in the discussion as an example of an article published in Science where the authors propose clonidine to reduce craving but evaluate using a question described as "thinking about cigarettes wish to smoke." Other authors wrote that "craving is the earliest, the most consistent, and the most severe symptom of tobacco withdrawal" [5].

Thinking that a person has stopped contact with an appetizing target (be it cigarettes or food), if this part of a frequency context, thoughts about it are expected to arise, which is not so simple to state is whether that would be craving, and what are the criteria for a cognitive and affective experience to be classified as a craving. Kozlowski and Wilkinson, in 1987, proposed four representations of craving in schematic form, highlighting the fourth proposal, as being:

1. Craving and symptoms constitute physical dependence (proposed by Jellinek)
2. Craving is one like many other symptoms (DSM III Tobacco Withdrawal Syndrome)
3. Craving is the result of physical symptoms (proposed by Marlatt)
4. Symptoms a) unconditioned or b) conditioned are the causers and also caused by cognitive craving processes that influence and are also influenced by external stimuli (Ludwig & Wikler).

Up to this point it seems that it was unclear whether craving was a subjective, behavioral, or physiological state. After this publication, Kozlowski and Wilkinson needed to write one more text positioning themselves in relation to all the responses they received from different authors [6]. They start with a first premise, that it is better to use the term craving when its use is more appropriate than the term desire, the authors argue that "Craving is a subset of desires which crosses a threshold of intensity." Another issue raised is the difference between intentions to use a substance and the desire to use it. The authors end their ideas with an excerpt that says: "In a scientific study of addictions, we think that the construct of 'craving' is one of the easiest to fool oneself with, and therefore suggest that investigators handle it with care" [6].

2. Understanding the Food Craving's Episode

When it comes to intense craving, in the old literature, one of the first studies found deals with the intense craving for non-food substances [7] which is little studied when considering Pica [8]. In 1962, the focus of a craving for food is described in the article entitled "To depression the craving for food" [9], and then publications considering the gestational and premenstrual period [10-12]. The framework of the vision of research on substance use was being replicated to eating behavior when craving is denoted as an aggravating factor, which represents a risk for consumption and, at the same time, something that must be controlled. Wardle in 1987 writes that "The phenomenology of compulsive eating encouraged comparisons with addictive behaviors" [13]. In the same way as saying that sexual desire depends only on hormone levels, reducing desire to just one dimension is unsatisfactory. Defining craving and FC seems challenging in face of so many research questions and hypotheses to define a construct, but clarity about the phenomenon seems to be an essential part of when obtaining an investigation. In Old English craving is derived from the term *crafian*, which means "to beg" [14].

Currently, the best definition, published in 2005, says that desire is "a cognitive event loaded with affectivity where an object or activity associated with pleasure or relief is in attentional focus." According to the authors, even carrying the content of affections, desire is distinguished from a simple emotion, as the conscious psychological experience includes images and verbal thoughts about the target's attractiveness and characteristics [15]. In this theory an important distinction between desires and their antecedents. Just as for food, the differentiation between hunger and desire is very clear, there is confusion in the self-report between desire and the associated cognitions (such as intentions) or difficulty in resisting thoughts [16], as their occurrence can increase the probability of desire, but they do not represent the desire itself. According to the authors, it is important to consider the occurrence of unconscious processes that can even trigger the desire (such as a small will, which is still unspecific) but which are not the desire itself. This goes against the theory of Robinson and Berridge who argue that, when cognitive elaboration consciously translates incentive salience attributions, there is activation of the "willing" system that contributed to the experience" [17]. From the point of view of eating behavior, the state called "I want to eat" may be a reflection of this still unconscious activation that will be orchestrated by the internal state such as the level of hunger, and then yes, "I want to eat because I'm hungry and so I want eat a specific food," this same example is valid for the presence of a specific desire in the absence of hunger, both being the desire for food, but when this desire is accompanied by a process of elaboration and awareness of lack and an increased negative deficit, the FC episode is characterized by a marked urgency for food consumption. Thus, the best insight of the theory proposed by is that if the intrusions cause significant pleasure or relief, cognitive elaborations usually occur, a process that increases the intensity and sense of urgency, where desire turns into craving [18]. And this process depends on an elaboration. The elaborations increase in number and intensity to the point of shifting the attentional focus, and this phenomenon occurs because there is a direction of information (like a food script) on how to reach or achieve the appetizing target that is being imagined. This event prioritizes a cognitive processing for the elaboration that occupies a space in the working memory [18]. The Elaborated Intrusion Theory of cravings argues that (1) psychological abstinence, (2) ambient associations, (3) cognitive, and (4) negative affect are potential triggers for cravings.

Something new for FC research is to identify parallel thoughts that conflict with the elaborations of desire, not the suppression of thoughts, well known in this process, but the thoughts of diet (or diet mentality), that is, the role of cognitive restriction as an opponent, which can increase awareness of the lack, but the need (rule or dietary belief) that this lack is necessary, as seen in dieters [19]. One of the sufferings mentioned during the diet, in addition to increased anxiety, is the intense desire for food (craving). Currently, there are some instruments developed to study this construct, such as: Food Craving Record, Visual Analog Scale (VAS) for Food Craving, Food Craving Inventory (FCI), Food Craving Questionnaire and Food Craving Questionnaire Trait and Stait (FCQ-T/S). The FCI was developed by White and collaborators (2002) and assesses the frequency of food craving in the previous month and generates a total score and four subscales (high fats, carbohydrates/starches, and fast-food fats) [20, 21].

3. Understanding the Triggers to Food Craving

Getting in touch with an external clue about food, such as viewing an advertisement, seeing an image on Instagram, or hearing someone talking about a food, can generate mental images of what it would be like to eat this food, what it would taste like, how it would smell, and the pleasure of consuming it. If the food has already been consumed on that day or within a close period, it is less likely to be desired, but it still exists. But in case that in recent times this suggested food has not been consumed, the probability of craving is greater. A feeling of enchantment and anticipation for consumption can generate awareness of lack, deprivation and how good it would be to consume this food. This thought captures attention, and images of how to achieve it, and how pleasurable it would be to have it invade the mind and accumulate in the working memory, which, at the same time, generates discomfort for lack and attentional focus on unconsummated pleasure. In short, several factors can be associated with the emergence or intensification of desires and FC.

Eating Disorders (ED) represent a specific target for understanding FC, as they are the population with higher levels when measured through questionnaires, VAS associated or not with experimental tasks. The analysis of the available literature over the last thirty years on ED resulted in the unification of 12 possible factors associated with FC. These are divided into two large dimensions, the external factors, related to the environment and configurations present in it and cultural associations, and the internal factors which relate to mental processes and physiological sensations that involve the regulation of food consumption, pleasure, and avoidant possibilities in relation to food.

In this chapter we will call triggers considering the occurrence of an elaboration process and the outcome of dysfunctional eating behavior such as emotional eating and binge eating. A relationship is given by increased FC intensity starting at lower levels for Anorexia Nervosa followed by Bulimia Nervosa and higher levels for Binge Eating Disorder [21, 22].

3.1. External Factors

3.1.1. Positive/Negative Events

It was also found that the time of day may be associated with FC. In the afternoon/early evening and in the late evening/night [23]. Also when the antecedent factors for binge eating were studied, Binge eating resulted from FC more often if the women were alone, in the morning, and following eating the craved food [24]. In another study, women with FC had higher ratings of boredom and anxiety during the day, and dysphoric mood was significantly present prior to the cravings [25].

3.1.2. Food Environment

Some authors point to the food environment as a major influence on food choices by creating an appetitive counterpart to the "psychological effects of other hedonically-driven activities" as suggested by some researchers [26]. Patients with BN/BED reported higher FC and anxiety levels across all food-related virtual environments than the non-clinical sample [27]. The term hedonic hunger has been used in this context considering the dichotomous division between homeostatic and non-homeostatic systems, and recently this view has been questioned [28, 29].

3.1.3. Advertising

The study of the effects of marketing on eating behavior has shown interaction mechanisms between increased interest and drive for consumption in the absence of energy needs [30], with many studies carried out in the childhood obesity scenario [31]. Studies show that some behaviors presented in advertisements are imitated, such as holding food, moving food to mouth, taking a bite, chewing on food affects consumers. In two studies, the authors found that the participants experienced an increased desire to eat the depicted food and they ate more of the advertised food when the model was shown to engage in eating food compared with when the model was shown during completion of a consumption episode [32]. Attentional biases and their relationship with impulsiveness have been demonstrated in this context for cases of people with obesity [33] and ED [34].

3.1.4. Cultural Beliefs about Food

Eating habits and foods can refer to a specific culture, and, be internalized in other cultures. There are several cultural evidence about it: Prevalence of cravings, frequency, types of food desired, and gender differences [35]. American women are twice as likely to have chocolate cravings as American men (91% vs. 59%). On the other hand, when men and women are compared in Spain, the prevalence is similar (90% vs. 78%) [36]. The word craving does not have an exact translation in some countries around the world, so the importance can be decreased [14].

Women may view menstruation as a socially sanctioned justification for indulging in a "taboo" food, resulting in a cyclical increase in reported craving frequency [37]. Women of diverse backgrounds (n = 275) reported frequency and triggers of desire and completed validated measures of acculturation. Foreign-born women were significantly less prone to menstrual cravings for chocolate compared to women born to US-born parents and second-generation immigrants [37]. When comparing differences between Argentina, Brazil, France, and USA, in all countries, men were more pro-meat, in free associations, taste, desire and consumption frequency. Brazil and Argentina were generally the most positive, followed by France and the United States [38]. For Japanese, rice is leading the ten most desired foods, leaving chocolate in second place [39]. The findings indicate that food desires are also a social construct. Food availability, symbolism and cultural norms are associated with cultural issues related to gender, life stage, nationality, and acculturation.

3.1.5. Specific Places

Studies using Virtual Reality (VR) in ED patients have shown several results that demonstrate the association between increased FC levels when these individuals are exposed to different types of environments, the environments being related to food consumption (e.g., kitchen and coffee shop). Also, increase of FC were produced in the kitchen, bedroom, dining room, and bakery situations [40, 41].

3.1.6. Food by Itself

BN/BED patients reported increase of FC and anxiety when exposed to virtual food than controls [42]. In another study the levels of FC increase after food exposure in patients with BED [43]. When controlling for baseline FC, chocolate pictures evoked an increase FC response than neutral pictures in participants [44]. Desire-related thoughts can also be induced through semantic cues or instructions, which can create an image of the appetitive target [45]. The subjective vividness of the images is strongly correlated with the intensity of desire [46]. According to a proposed model, the exposure to highly palatable foods can lead to anticipation of the risk of overeating and increase the anxiety experienced [47].

3.2. Internal Factors

3.2.1. Dietary Restriction

Models for the etiology of ED have already described dietary restriction as a trigger for binge eating. In the ED, although some food choices are preferably from the food repertoire, the momentary reward is prioritized and focused on the moment rather than considering the possibility of an adjustment in the food day and week (which would be unacceptable from the point of view of food beliefs). Thinking about possibilities of control, and dietary changes can evoke a feeling of deprivation, and dissatisfaction ("I feel fat," thought about the body) or ("I need to eat less chocolate," thought about diet). Some types of thoughts involve the desire for food, and because of their characteristic of composing eating attitudes, they can increase the probability of consumption. Thus, dietary restrictions are carried out from a cognitive as well as a behavioral point of view (i.e., dietary restriction). The predominant emotional reaction in many episodes of desire is negative because negative emotion is a potential precursor to desire and a consequence of it [18]. Both are associated with the arise and maintenance of binge eating, but in cases of anorexia of the restrictive subtype (marked by inflexibility and other neural changes) the restriction is maintained, and FC levels are the lowest compared to other diagnoses [22, 48, 49].

3.2.2. Food Reward

The use of the term food reward is related to what is compensated, which is reciprocated, to repair damage. In eating behavior, it is an eating conditioned to a situation or belief "I ate to reward myself." From a neuroscience point of view, the reward is any object or event that produces an approaching behavior and makes us devote energy and attention to it. Patients with BN/BED exhibited decrease activation in Posterior cingulate cortex (PCC), during the anticipation of food reward and increase activation in PCC, medial Orbitofrontal cortex and anterior medial Prefrontal cortex during the receipt of food reward [50]. Women whit binge-type ED endorse higher FC, eating for purposes of copying, and eating for purposes of reward enhancement [51]. Obese men (n = 9) received a moderate dose (0.5 mg/kg) or high dose (1.0 mg/kg) of methylphenidate, a dopamine reuptake inhibitor (which increases the availability of brain dopamine) or placebo. Afterwards, participants were instructed to consume the desired amount of pizza. As a result, there was a 23% reduction in the moderate dose group, and a 43% reduction in the high dose group [52].

3.2.3. Impulsiveness/Inflexibility

Behavioral drives for palatable foods are moderated by cognition, specifically executive functions. These mental functions support self-regulation of eating behavior [53]. From a neural and neuropsychological point of view, many advances have shown differences between diagnoses [54], with AN cases being marked with inflexibility and associated with lower FC levels [22] while BN/BED are marked by difficulty in controlling impulses [21]. In many moments, food comes as a condition and not a choice. Inattentive and/or emotional eating and binge eating or eating very restricted could be conditions, all examples of a disconnection with the real need and desire. These aspects will be related to specific thoughts and beliefs about food. Restrictive eaters will have a greater chance of losing control [55].

3.2.4. Emotions, Thoughts, and Feelings about Food

Throughout the development of eating habits, we like and want some specific foods, and this relates to (1) exposure to food, (2) context of consumption, and (3) individual preferences [56, 57].

Eating attitudes are composed of emotions, feelings, and thoughts about food, and these can influence behavior (action, consumption) [58, 59]. Diet thoughts or thoughts related to food self-control are the basis of cognitive restriction that can lead the individual to enter in caloric restriction or to think about ways to enter restriction, thus eating with intentions of cognitive restriction. It may also involve dysfunctional eating beliefs that were culturally learned or based on associations of eating habits construction. For patients with BN an improvement in mood after the fasting period was demonstrated, which goes against the behavioral reinforcers seen in the psychopathology of BN, despite the increase in FC to the simultaneous detriment [60]. The subscales 'desire' and 'lack of control' of the FC questionnaires have been shown to be positively associated with eating and weight concerns (EDE-Q), and 'lack of control' is inversely correlated with shape concerns [61].

3.2.5. Hunger/Satiety/Appetite

Being hungry and a negative mood was also strongly associated with FC [23]. For BED patients had increased FC scores for pre and post exposure to food compared to Obese and normal-weight controls; The levels of hunger was no difference between groups, but patients with BED consumed significant more [43].

3.2.6. Anxious/Depressive Symptoms

Emotional dysregulation is associated with the emergence of FC as forms of relief, through emotional eating, which can become compulsive eating given other trigger associations such as the presence of dietary restriction through fasting or restrictive diet. Treatment with Repetitive transcranial magnetic stimulation (RTMS) has shown good results for markers related to anxiety and depressive symptoms. Salivary cortisol concentrations following real RTMS were significantly lower compared with those following sham RTMS [62].

Another study showed decrease in the FC levels in the subjective ratings of want to eat, urge to eat, and sense of hunger for the high-calorie food stimuli was found at post-RTMS session [63].

Although an episode of binge eating can occur regardless of the presence of a FC episode, the emotion regulation model [64] demonstrates many of the factors and their associations, seen as triggers for the occurrence of an outcome such as binge eating. The occurrence of a negative event (factor 3.1.1 - Positive/negative events) such as receiving a criticism from the boss (Angela's model of binge eating [64]), was associated with the emergence of a negative emotional state with feelings of anger, hurt and shame that was followed by an attempt to escape from the emotional experience (factor 3.3.4 - Emotions/Thoughts/Feelings about food). This attempt to escape may be associated with the appearance of FC, when Angela stops at the cafeteria and has a binge eating as described in the model. Recently, two situations related to emotional eating were described in a qualitative study, 1) experiencing negative emotions, with ensuing FC; and 2) after losing control to emotional eating, with ensuing feelings of low self-esteem [65], and dialectical coaching strategies were used.

Another proposed model puts as an initial trigger to smell, to see and to feel the food (factor 3.2.1 - Food itself), which culminated in an intense desire (followed by guilt and disappointment). In this case, the conflict between the experience and elaboration of the desire with the thoughts that generate the feeling of guilt and disappointment for the desire (factor 3.3.4 - Emotions/Thoughts/Feelings about food). In this case, Leticia's example described in the book states that the attempt to escape the emotional experience was made with food consumption (factor 3.3.7 - Food reward) which triggered a binge eating. These and several other aspects place the (1) factors in association (in the absence of FC) and the (2) emergence of FC in response to the associated factors as conditions for compulsive eating behavior, bringing greater clarity to the individual description of the characteristics of a clinical condition and for its future therapeutic proposal.

4. Now That I Can Eat Everything, I Don't Want to Eat All the Time: The Effect of Unconditional Permission to Eat on Food Cravings

The discussion about the need to understand FC instead of trying to control it is recent [66], but only a non-moralizing view on FC can open possibilities for interventions that do not increase the unacceptability of desires. The process of restricting foods in a diet is facilitated by components of cognitive restriction - thoughts and attitudes towards decreasing consumption - and behavioral aspects (decreasing food consumption) [67, 68]. Cognitive restriction may have associations with beliefs and cognitive distortions that are all the time being spread, reinforced by lifestyle and dietary groups. As dieting is currently representative of symbolism and lifestyle. Those who follow a lifestyle that includes a restrictive diet generate a phenomenon of differentiation with a series of meanings attributed to food consumption that distance the simple eater from a dieter [69].

Thus, aspects related to commensality are reconfigured, with the abandon of eating to socialize in exchange for isolation or grouping among those who are similar. Despite the increase in evidence and specific recommendations, contemporary food has been demarcated by three points highlighted by Mayes & Thompson, such as (1) the simplification of this science to increase the persuasion of dietary orientation, (2) superficial references that justify ideological views and (3) the presumption that nutrition is the primary value of food. These are initial aspects related to the view that an individual may desire food [71].

4.1. Meanings of Food and Its Relationship with Desire

Thus, food desires often enter a food context that reflects improvisation or something "off plan." Also, when the desired foods come in by condition, such as emotional eating, reinforcing the consumption of a tasty food in moments where there is negative affect (and the desire for relief), thus, overall, there is dissatisfaction with food.

Currently, the view that one has of the treatment of eating behavior puts control in valorization and disregards several factors that are involved in the emergence of FC. An example of this aspect is a recent review where the authors point out that "Being able to control food cravings is a determinant of success at adhering to an energy-restricted diet regimen" [72]. Many of the strategies even involve the use of medications, which could benefit from integration with nutritional treatment aimed at understanding FC [66] and not their control. Some problematic issues can be raised, such as excessive cognitive control, and directed to some foods, as in the example of cognitive restriction [73], which can generate a greater sense of guilt linked to the onset of FC, that is, when disregarding whether the components of eating behavior and therapeutic actions can generate unsustainable long-term results.

One of the insights initially based on science, and now proven through several studies [74-78] is the Intuitive Eating approach, which starts from three great principles that lead to food satisfaction, they are (1) A unconditional permission to eat, (2) Eating more for physical reasons than emotional, and (3) Tuning to the inner signals of hunger and satiety [79]. All these factors can be worked on in the absence of a need for dietary self-control. Probably whoever controls himself, will get out of control, so it is necessary to integrate the internal state, as seen for the factors that influence FC, such as External: (1) Positive/negative events; (2) Food environment; (3) Advertisements; (4) Cultural beliefs about food; (5) Specific locations and (6) Food for itself, Internal factors: (7) Dietary restriction, (8) Food reward; (9) Impulsiveness/Inflexibility; (10) Emotions, thoughts and feelings about food; (11) Hunger/satiation/ appetite and (12) Anxious/depressive symptoms.

While craving levels need to be elevated for AN cases, in cases of AN binge/purge subtype, BN and BED and Disordered Eating, FC levels are related to negative outcomes such as binge eating. The challenge for treatment is the use of cognitive-behavioral strategies associated with

Intuitive Eating principles to regulate and bring about food awareness. Strategies related to Mindfulness and Mindful Eating have been associated with FC decrease, that is, practices and principles not related to control [80-83]. These strategies and practices can promote the satisfaction of FC and a decrease in FC, as predicted by the Intuitive Eating, but when the focus of interventions is only on reducing body weight, a moralistic view can be used by professionals, or maintained as basis of thought and way of dealing with the food of the individual who is being treated. Sociocultural and identity aspects are part of a good treatment of eating behavior, and these may include questioning established cultural beliefs regarding body and food [84, 85], and acceptance-based approaches to the management of craving [86].

Conclusion

Several advances in the understanding of desires and FC have been made in recent years, with emphasis on the important role that FCs play in outcomes of eating behavior. In addition to the negative outcomes already known in eating disorder behavior, there is still little literature on specific tests of how FC levels behave in response to nutritional treatment of specific populations and what approaches would be related to their improvement, both from a nutritional point of view, as well as a psychological one. As a challenge, to consider the approaches of self-control and those related to self-regulation based on recent findings and developments within the evolution of practices in psychology. Nutritional approaches related to eating behavior are still scarce and little used, as well as protocol proposals in different clinical and cultural contexts.

References

[1] Weingarten HP, Elston D. The phenomenology of food cravings. *Appetite* 1990; 15: 231-246.

[2] Ludwig AM, Wikler A. " Craving" and relapse to drink. *Q. J. Stud. Alcohol.* 1974; 35: 108-130.

[3] Ludwig AM, Wikler A, Stark LH. The first drink: Psychobiological aspects of craving. *Arch. Gen. Psychiatry* 1974; 30: 539-547.

[4] Kozlowski LT, Wilkinson DA. Use and misuse of the concept of craving by alcohol, tobacco, and drug researchers. *Br. J. Addict.* 1987; 82: 31-45.

[5] Glassman AH, Jackson WK, Walsh BT, et al. Cigarette craving, smoking withdrawal, and clonidine. *Science* 1984; 226: 864-866.

[6] Kozlowski LT, Wilkinson DA. Comments on Kozlowski & *Wilkinson's "Use and misuse of the concept of craving by alcohol, tobacco and drug researchers": A reply from the authors.*

[7] Snapper I. Food preferences in man: special cravings and aversions. *Ann. N. Y. Acad. Sci.* 1955; 63: 92-106.

[8] Oliveira J de, Cordás TA. Eating behavior, non-food substance consumption and negative urgency in women. *Einstein (São Paulo)* 2020; 18: eAO5269.

[9] Stuart DM. To depress the craving for food. *Am. J. Nurs.* 1962; 62: 88-92.

[10] Dickens G, Trethowan WH. Cravings and aversions during pregnancy. *J. Psychosom. Res.* 1971; 15: 259-268.

[11] Marcus RL. Cravings for food in pregnancy. *Manch. Med. Gaz.* 1965; 44: 16-17.

[12] Smith SL, Sauder C. Food cravings, depression, and premenstrual problems. *Psychosom. Med.* 1969; 31: 281-287.

[13] Wardle J. Compulsive eating and dietary restraint. *Br. J. Clin. Psychol.* 1987; 26: 47-55.

[14] Hormes JM, Rozin P. Does "craving" carve nature at the joints? Absence of a synonym for craving in many languages. *Addict. Behav.* 2010; 35: 459-463.

[15] Salkovskis PM, Reynolds M. Thought suppression and smoking cessation. *Behav. Res. Ther.* 1994; 32: 193-201.

[16] Tiffany ST, Singleton E, Haertzen CA, et al. The development of a cocaine craving questionnaire. *Drug Alcohol Depend.* 1993; 34: 19-28.

[17] Robinson TE, Berridge KC. Addiction. *Annu. Rev. Psychol.* 2003; 54: 25-53.

[18] Kavanagh DJ, Andrade J, May J. Imaginary relish and exquisite torture: The elaborated intrusion theory of desire. *Psychol. Rev.* 2005; 112: 446-467.

[19] Foreyt JP, Goodrick GK. *Living without dieting*. Harrison Publishing, 1992.

[20] White MA, Whisenhunt BL, Williamson DA, et al. Development and validation of the food-craving inventory. *Obes. Res.* 2002; 10: 107-114.

[21] Oliveira J, Cordás TA. The body asks and the mind judges: Food cravings in eating disorders. *Encephale*. Epub ahead of print 2020. doi: https://doi.org/10.1016/j.encep.2020.01.003.

[22] Moreno S, Warren CS, Rodriguez S, et al. Food cravings discriminate between anorexia and bulimia nervosa. Implications for "success" versus "failure" in dietary restriction. *Appetite* 2009; 52: 588-594.

[23] Ferrer-Garcia M, Gutierrez-Maldonado J, Agliaro-Lopez M, et al. Validation of VR-based Software for Binge Eating Treatment: Preliminary Data. *Stud. Health Technol. Inform.* 2014; 199: 146-150.

[24] Waters A, Hill A, Waller G. Internal and external antecedents of binge eating episodes in a group of women with bulimia nervosa. *Int. J. Eat Disord.* 2001; 29: 17-22.

[25] Hill AJ, Weaver CF, Blundell JE. Food craving, dietary restraint and mood. *Appetite* 1991; 17: 187-197.

[26] Lowe MR, Butryn ML. Hedonic hunger: A new dimension of appetite? *Physiol. Behav.* 2007; 91: 432-439.

[27] Pla-Sanjuanelo J, Ferrer-Garcia M, Vilalta-Abella F, et al. VR-based cue-exposure therapy (VR-CET) versus VR-CET plus

pharmacotherapy in the treatment of bulimic-type eating disorders. *Annu. Rev. Cybertherapy Telemed.* 2017; 15: 116-122.

[28] Aston-Jones G, Smith RJ, Sartor GC, et al. Lateral hypothalamic orexin/hypocretin neurons: A role in reward-seeking and addiction. *Brain Res.* 2010; 1314: 74-90.

[29] Sternson SM, Eiselt A-K. Three pillars for the neural control of appetite. *Annu. Rev. Physiol.* 2017; 79: 401-423.

[30] Harris JL, Pomeranz JL, Lobstein T, et al. A crisis in the marketplace: how food marketing contributes to childhood obesity and what can be done. *Annu. Rev. Public Health* 2009; 30: 211-225.

[31] Norman J, Kelly B, McMahon A-T, et al. Remember Me? Exposure to Unfamiliar Food Brands in Television Advertising and Online Advergames Drives Children's Brand Recognition, Attitudes, and Desire to Eat Foods: A Secondary Analysis from a Crossover Experimental-Control Study with Randomization at the Group Level. *J. Acad. Nutr. Diet.* 2020; 120: 120-129.

[32] Palcu J, Haasova S, Florack A. Advertising models in the act of eating: How the depiction of different eating phases affects consumption desire and behavior. *Appetite* 2019; 139: 59-66.

[33] Bongers P, van de Giessen E, Roefs A, et al. Being impulsive and obese increases susceptibility to speeded detection of high-calorie foods. *Heal Psychol. Off J. Div. Heal Psychol. Am. Psychol. Assoc.* 2015; 34: 677-685.

[34] Reents J, Pedersen A. Differences in Food Craving in Individuals With Obesity With and Without Binge Eating Disorder. *Front. Psychol.* 2021; 12: 2112.

[35] Orloff NC, Flammer A, Hartnett J, et al. Food cravings in pregnancy: Preliminary evidence for a role in excess gestational weight gain. *Appetite* 2016; 105: 259-265.

[36] Osman JL, Sobal J. Chocolate cravings in American and Spanish individuals: biological and cultural influences. *Appetite* 2006; 47: 290-301.

[37] Hormes JM, Niemiec MA. Does culture create craving? Evidence from the case of menstrual chocolate craving. *PLoS One* 2017; 12: e0181445.

[38] Ruby MB, Alvarenga MS, Rozin P, et al. Attitudes toward beef and vegetarians in Argentina, Brazil, France, and the USA. *Appetite* 2016; 96: 546-554.

[39] Komatsu S. Rice and sushi cravings: a preliminary study of food craving among Japanese females. *Appetite* 2008; 50: 353-358.

[40] Pla-Sanjuanelo J, Ferrer-Garcia M, Gutierrez-Maldonado J, et al. Identifying specific cues and contexts related to bingeing behavior for the development of effective virtual environments. *Appetite* 2015; 87: 81-89.

[41] Pla-Sanjuanelo J, Ferrer-Garcia M, Gutiérrez-Maldonado J, et al. Trait and State Craving as Indicators of Validity of VR-based Software for Binge Eating Treatment. *Stud. Health Technol. Inform.* 2015; 219: 141-146.

[42] Ferrer-Garcia M, Pla-Sanjuanelo J, Dakanalis A, et al. Eating behavior style predicts craving and anxiety experienced in food-related virtual environments by patients with eating disorders and healthy controls. *Appetite* 2017; 117: 284-293.

[43] Ng L, Davis C. Cravings and food consumption in binge eating disorder. *Eat. Behav.* 2013; 14: 472-475.

[44] Wolz I, Granero R, Fernández-Aranda F. A comprehensive model of food addiction in patients with binge-eating symptomatology: The essential role of negative urgency. *Compr. Psychiatry* 2017; 74: 118-124.

[45] Cepeda-Benito A, Tiffany ST. The use of a dual-task procedure for the assessment of cognitive effort associated with cigarette craving. *Psychopharmacology (Berl)* 1996; 127: 155-163.

[46] Tiffany ST, Drobes DJ. Imagery and smoking urges: the manipulation of affective content. *Addict. Behav.* 1990; 15: 531-539.

[47] Schyns G, Roefs A, Mulkens S, et al. Expectancy violation, reduction of food cue reactivity and less eating in the absence of

hunger after one food cue exposure session for overweight and obese women. *Behav. Res. Ther.* 2016; 76: 57-64.
[48] Gendall KA, Sullivan PF, Joyce PR, et al. Food cravings in women with a history of anorexia nervosa. *Int. J. Eat. Disord.* 1997; 22: 403-409.
[49] Veenstra EM, de Jong PJ. Reduced Automatic Motivational Orientation Towards Food in Restricting Anorexia Nervosa. *J. Abnorm. Psychol.* 2011; 120: 708-718.
[50] Simon JJ, Skunde M, Walther S, et al. Neural signature of food reward processing in bulimic-type eating disorders. *Soc. Cogn. Affect. Neurosci.* 2016; 11: 1393-1401.
[51] Leslie M, Turton R, Burgess E, et al. Testing the addictive appetite model of binge eating: The importance of craving, coping, and reward enhancement. *Eur. Eat. Disord. Rev.* 2018; 26: 541-550.
[52] Leddy JJ, Epstein LH, Jaroni JL, et al. Influence of methylphenidate on eating in obese men. *Obes. Res.* 2004; 12: 224-232.
[53] Meye FJ, Adan RAH. Feelings about food: The ventral tegmental area in food reward and emotional eating. *Trends Pharmacol. Sci.* 2014; 35: 31-40.
[54] Kaye WH, Wierenga CE, Bailer UF, et al. Nothing tastes as good as skinny feels: The neurobiology of anorexia nervosa. *Trends Neurosci.* 2013; 36: 110-120.
[55] Eldredge KL. An investigation of the influence of dieting and self-esteem on dietary disinhibition. *Int. J. Eat. Disord.* 1993; 13: 57-67.
[56] Sobal J, Bisogni CA. Constructing food choice decisions. *Ann. Behav. Med.*; 38. Epub ahead of print 2009. doi: 10.1007/s12160-009-9124-5.
[57] Rogers PJ, Smit HJ. Food craving and food “addiction”: a critical review of the evidence from a biopsychosocial perspective. *Pharmacol. Biochem. Behav.* 2000; 66: 3-14.
[58] Katz D, Stotland E. A preliminary statement to a theory of attitude structure and change. *Psychol. A study a Sci.*; 3.

[59] Eiger MR, Christie BW, Sucher KP. Changing in eating attitudes: An outcome measure of patients with eating disorders. *J. Acad. Nutr. Diet.* 1996; 96: 62.

[60] Moreno-Domínguez S, Rodríguez-Ruiz S, Fernández-Santaella MC, et al. Impact of fasting on food craving, mood and consumption in bulimia nervosa and healthy women participants. *Eur. Eat. Disord. Rev.* 2012; 20: 461-467.

[61] Van den Eynde F, Koskina A, Syrad H, et al. State and trait food craving in people with bulimic eating disorders. *Eat. Behav.* 2012; 13: 414-417.

[62] Claudino AM, Van den Eynde F, Stahl D, et al. Repetitive transcranial magnetic stimulation reduces cortisol concentrations in bulimic disorders. *Psychol. Med.* 2011; 41: 1329-1336.

[63] Sutoh C, Koga Y, Kimura H, et al. Repetitive Transcranial Magnetic Stimulation Changes Cerebral Oxygenation on the Left Dorsolateral Prefrontal Cortex in Bulimia Nervosa: A Near-Infrared Spectroscopy Pilot Study. *Eur. Eat. Disord. Rev.* 2016; 24: 83-88.

[64] Safer DL, Adler S, Masson PC. *The DBT? Solution for Emotional Eating: A Proven Program to Break the Cycle of Bingeing and Out-of-Control Eating*. Guilford Publications, 2018.

[65] Dol A, Bode C, Velthuijsen H, et al. Application of three different coaching strategies through a virtual coach for people with emotional eating: a vignette study. *J. Eat. Disord.* 2021; 9: 1-15.

[66] Oliveira J, Cordás TA. Should Food Cravings be Controlled or Understood? *J. Exp. Neurol.*; 1.

[67] Richardson AS, Arsenault JE, Cates SC, et al. Perceived stress, unhealthy eating behaviors, and severe obesity in low-income women. *Nutr. J.* 2015; 14: 122.

[68] Banna JC, Panizza CE, Boushey CJ, et al. Association between Cognitive Restraint, Uncontrolled Eating, Emotional Eating and BMI and the Amount of Food Wasted in Early Adolescent Girls. *Nutrients*; 10. Epub ahead of print September 2018. doi: 10.3390/nu 10091279.

[69] Pellerano JA, Gimenes-Minasse MHSG. "Low Carb, High Fat": Comensalidade E Sociabilidade Em Tempos De Dietas Restritivas [Commensality and sociability in times of restrictive diets]. *DEMETRA Aliment Nutr. Saúde* [DEMETRA Food Nutr. Health] 2015; 10: 493-506.

[70] Azevedo E de. Liberem a Dieta [release the diet]. *DEMETRA Aliment Nutr Saúde* [*DEMETRA Food Nutr. Health*] 2015; 10: 717-728.

[71] Mayes CR, Thompson DB. What Should We Eat? Biopolitics, Ethics, and Nutritional Scientism. *J. Bioeth. Inq.* 2015; 12: 587-599.

[72] Rebello CJ, Greenway FL. Reward-Induced Eating: Therapeutic Approaches to Addressing Food Cravings. *Adv. Ther.* 2016; 33: 1853-1866.

[73] Oliveira J, Colombarolli MS, Figueredo LS, et al. Cognitive restraint directed at carbohydrates in individuals on low-carb diet with binge eating: the role of guilt about food cravings. *Einstein (São Paulo)*; 19.

[74] Cadena-Schlam L, López-Guimerà G. Ingesta intuitiva: Un nuevo abordaje del comportamiento alimentario [Intuitive Eating: A New Approach to Eating Behavior]. *Nutr. Hosp.* 2015; 31: 995-1002.

[75] Homan KJ, Tylka TL. Development and exploration of the gratitude model of body appreciation in women. *Body Image* 2018; 25: 14-22.

[76] Warren JM, Smith N, Ashwell M. Effectiveness and associated potential mechanisms. *Nutr. Res. Rev.* 2017; 30: 272-283.

[77] Webber KH, Mellin L, Mayes L, et al. Pilot Investigation of 2 Nondiet Approaches to Improve Weight and Health. *Altern. Ther. Health Med.* 2018; 24: 16-20.

[78] Wilson RE, Marshall RD, Murakami JM, et al. Brief non-dieting intervention increases intuitive eating and reduces dieting intention, body image dissatisfaction, and anti-fat attitudes: A randomized controlled trial. *Appetite* 2020; 148: 104556.

[79] Tribole E, Resch E. *Intuitive eating: A revolutionary anti-diet approach*. St. Martin's Essentials, 2020.

[80] Dunn C, Haubenreiser M, Johnson M, et al. Mindfulness Approaches and Weight Loss, Weight Maintenance, and Weight Regain. *Curr. Obes. Rep.* 2018; 7: 37-49.

[81] Jenkins KT, Tapper K. Resisting chocolate temptation using a brief mindfulness strategy. *Br. J. Health Psychol.* 2014; 19: 509-522.

[82] Tapper K, Turner A. The effect of a mindfulness-based decentering strategy on chocolate craving. *Appetite* 2018; 130: 157-162.

[83] Tapper K. Mindfulness and craving: effects and mechanisms. *Clin. Psychol. Rev.* 2018; 59: 101-117.

[84] Satter E. Eating competence: Nutrition education with the Satter eating competence model. *J. Nutr. Educ. Behav.* 2007; 39: S189-S194.

[85] Krall JS, Lohse B. Validation of a measure of the Satter eating competence model with low-income females. *Int. J. Behav. Nutr. Phys. Act* 2011; 8: 1-10.

[86] Coffino JA, Heiss S, Hormes JM. Targeting acceptance in the management of food craving: The mediating roles of eating styles and thought suppression. *Eat. Behav.* 2018; 29: 132-136.

In: A Closer Look at Women's Health ISBN: 978-1-68507-408-1
Editor: Lakisha Roberts

Chapter 6

PHYSICAL ACTIVITY AS A TREATMENT STRATEGY DURING MENOPAUSAL TRANSITION - AN EVOLUTIONARY APPROACH

Sylvia Kirchengast*

Department of Evolutionary Anthropology,
University of Vienna, Vienna, Austria

ABSTRACT

Physical activity during menopausal transition is a recommended strategy to reduce climacteric complaints, to prevent obesity, metabolic and cardiovascular diseases but also to avoid accelerated bone loss resulting in long term health hazards such as osteoporosis. The positive effects of physical activity for the prevention of obesity, metabolic and cardiovascular diseases as well as an accelerated reduction of bone density are widely accepted. The effects of physical activity on climacteric symptomatology however, are controversially discussed. From an evolutionary viewpoint, we are designed to be physically

* Corresponding Author's E-mail: Sylvia.kirchengast@univie.ac.at.

active. Therefore, physical activity is not only a treatment strategy, it should be an essential part of our life. The present review focuses on the association between physical activity and menopausal transition from the viewpoint of evolutionary biology and evolutionary medicine.

Keywords: menopausal transition, physical activity, climacteric syndrome, sarcopenia, osteoporosis, health related quality of life, human evolution, evolutionary medicine

INTRODUCTION

Menopausal transition, commonly taking place between 40 and 60 years, is an important indicator of female reproductive senescence (Leidy-Sievert 2006; Gold 2011). The major event of menopausal transition is menopause itself, which biomedically is defined as the cessation of menstrual function and the irreversible termination of female reproductive capability, identified in retrospect after 12 months of amenorrhea (Lumdsen 2016). The ongoing trend of increasing life expectancy results not only in an increasing portion of elderly people in nearly all populations, but in particular, in an increase of menopausal and postmenopausal women, worldwide. About 25 million women experience menopause worldwide every year (Bojar et al. 2016). It is predicted, that we can expect more than 1.2 billon postmenopausal women worldwide in 2030.

Menopausal transition and postmenopause are associated with an increased risk of cardiovascular and metabolic diseases, but also with the various somatic and psychic symptoms of the climacteric syndrome (Woods 2005). Both conditions make menopausal transition and postmenopause uncomfortable for affected women and may reduce their health-related quality of life drastically. Menopausal women however, have important roles in their families but also in society and economy, consequently, climacteric complaints are perceived as especially stressful. Adequate strategies to reduce health risks associated with menopause and enhance quality of life of affected women are of special importance. Currently, beside hormone replacement therapy (HRT), several alternative treatment strategies are discussed to avoid menopause associated diseases and enhance health related quality of life. The present review focuses on the role of physical activity as a treatment strategy from the viewpoint of evolutionary biology and evolutionary medicine.

MENOPAUSE – DISEASE OR BIOLOGICAL PART OF FEMALE LIFE HISTORY

Menopause signifies the irreversible end of female reproductive function. Physiologically, menopause is the result of follicular atresia which starts during the fifth months of fetal development and continues until menopausal transition (Wu et al. 2005). During premenopause and menopausal transition, oocyte and follicular depletion accelerates. The reduction of follicle cells enhances the hormonal transition typical of this phase of life. Estrogen levels drop down because the aromatization of androgens to estrogens in the granulosa cells declines. This results in a severe alteration of the hypothalamic-pituitary-gonad axis. The low estrogen levels are detected by the hypothalamus resulting in an increased secretion of gonadotropin-releasing hormone (GnRH) there (Burger et al. 2007). Higher levels of GnRh force the pituitary gland to increase the secretion of the gonadotrophins FSH and LH, which should increase follicular maturation and estrogen synthesis in the granulosa cells of the ovaries. The depletion of oocytes and follicles however, prevent estrogen synthesis. As a consequence, the negative feedback mechanism of the HPG axis enhance GnRH and FSH as well as LH secretion. Therefore, the hormonal characteristic of menopausal transition and postmenopause are elevated FSH, but low estrogen levels (Burger et al. 2007).

All human females who live beyond the age of about 50 years undergo these hormonal alterations and experience the end of reproductive function (Leidy-Sievert 2006, Kirchengast & Rühli 2013).

Consequently, menopausal transition and menopause itself are not pathologies, and menopause is a natural part of female life history. Nevertheless, menopausal transition and the associated symptoms are mainly interpreted as pathologies, requiring medical treatment. This medicalization of menopause dated back in the 19th century, when the British gynecologist E.J. Tilt introduced menopause as a pathological condition in British Gynecology in 1857 (McCrea 1983; Van de Wiel 2014). In the 1930s, the interpretation of menopause as a disease was widely found in continental Europe and North America. Improvements in endocrinology and the availability of synthetic estrogens as medication resulted in the interpretation of menopause as a hormone deficiency disease in the 1960s (McCrea 1983; Van de Wiel 2014). As a consequence, the medical (pathological) viewpoint dominates menopause research for a long time.

Indeed, estrogen deficiency during menopausal transition and postmenopause is strongly associated with the appearance of the so-called climacteric syndrome, which reduces health related quality of life of affected women dramatically (Davies et al. 2015). All over the world and independent of culture, menopause is associated with a cluster of somatic symptoms such as hot flushes and night sweats but also vaginal dryness and psychic problems such as depression, irritability or insomnia. It is assumed, that up to 85% of postmenopausal women experience one or more climacteric symptoms during menopausal transition and postmenopause (Susmann et al. 2015; Woods 2005). In western societies, 60 to 70% of menopausal women reported severe climacteric complaints, first of all vasomotor symptoms (Palacios et.al. 2010, Monteleone et al. 2018). This symptom complex including vasomotor, urogenital but also psychic complaints, is commonly called climacteric syndrome, and seems to be strongly related to the menopause associated decline of estrogen levels (Burger et al. 2007). However, not all climacteric women suffer from climacteric symptoms and the interpretation of the individual symptoms varies between individuals but also according to culture and society (Beyene et al. 1986; Melby et al. 2005; Palacios et al. 2010).

Nevertheless, menopause is interpreted as an endocrinopathy and in particular, as an estrogen deficiency syndrome.

A quite different medical approach identifies menopause not as an own disease but as an important risk factor for other diseases. Epidemiological evidence shows that perimenopause and postmenopause are associated with an increased prevalence of various non-communicable diseases (Froehle 2013). Menopause associated estrogen deficiency accelerates bone loss and enhances the risk of osteoporosis, which represents a major public health problem (Tella et al. 2014). Furthermore, the decline of estrogen levels increases the risk of cardiovascular disease such as heart failure, hypertension but also stroke, metabolic syndrome, insulin resistance, type 2 diabetes (Stachowiak et al. 2015; Pu et al. 2018). In addition, somatic changes such as weight gain, obesity but also body composition changes, such as particular alterations of body fat distribution occur during this phase of life (Kirchengast et al. 1997). The progredient change from a gynoid fat distribution, typical of fertile phase towards a more android kind of fat patterning, characterized by a higher amount of adipose tissue at the abdominal region, has dramatic consequences for health and disease. An android fat distribution is significantly associated with an increased risk of the metabolic syndrome, cardiovascular disease and cancer (Lukacs et al. 2019). These menopause-associated changes in fat patterning are the result of the reduction in circulating levels of estrogens, in particular, 17β-estradiol. Consequently, the menopause associated decline of estrogen levels represents a marked risk factor for poor health and reduced health related quality of life among menopausal and postmenopausal women (Woods 2005). Therefore, the medical model of menopausal transition interprets the female body as poorly equipped to maintain normal metabolic function in the low-estrogen physiological environment after menopause (Austad 1997).

During the last century, human life expectancy increased dramatically, due to improvements in medicine, economy, sanitation and hygiene. As a consequence, the number of postmenopausal women increases worldwide every year, and a steadily increasing number of women is suffering from the decrease of estrogen levels and the associated climacteric symptomatology, but also other menopause associated health risks. Considering menopause as a hormone deficiency disease -as proposed by the medical model - hormone replacement therapy (HRT) was seen as the ideal strategy to replace lost estrogens and reduce in this way climacteric symptoms and other associated health risks (Fait 2019). In recent years however, the HRT has been increasingly criticized. HRT was interpreted as unnatural, and according to the results of the Women´s Health Initiative (WHI) and the Million Women Study, HRT increases the risk of cardiovascular disease and breast cancer (Narod 2011). Consequently, there is trend towards the use of alternative treatment strategies to reduce climacteric symptomology and estrogen decline associated health risks, but also to enhance well-being and health related quality of life during menopausal transition and postmenopause. One of these alternative treatment strategies was physical activity.

Physical Activity as a Treatment Strategy

Physical activity is a widely used strategy to enhance health and reduce the risk of chronic disease and disability (Pettree et al. 2015), but also to increase health related quality of life from early childhood up to old age (Sheikholeslami et al. 2018). With increasing age, a lack of physical activity seems to be associated with a progredient decrease of bone mass and bone density resulting in osteoporosis but also with a dramatic decrease of skeletal muscle mass resulting in sarcopenia (Kirchengast & Huber 2012). Both conditions are interrelated and increase the risk of developing the so-called frailty syndrome, which reduces not only health related quality of life, but also increases the risk to experience fatal bone fractures, such as of the femur neck and consequently, the risk of permanent invalidity and mortality (Kirchengast & Huber 2012).

Recently, the impact of physical activity as an alternative treatment strategy, on the especially vulnerable phase of female life cycle, the menopausal transition, was discussed. As mentioned above, physical activity is increasingly mentioned as an alternative therapy concept, to avoid accelerated bone loss and a reduction of skeletal muscle mass, to reduce the risk of metabolic and cardiovascular diseases and which might be suitable to reduce the degree of severity of climacteric symptoms (Nelson et al. 2007, 2008; Kim et al. 2014; Drabowska-Galas 2019). These positive effects on the climacteric syndrome however, is discussed controversial (Daley et al. 2007; 2015). A poorly discussed approach to explain the effects of physical activity on well-being and health during menopausal transition and beyond is an evolutionary one. On the one hand, the importance of sufficient physical activity can be interpreted from the viewpoint of evolutionary biology and in particular within the framework of human evolution. On the other hand, physical activity as a treatment strategy can be discussed from the viewpoint of Evolutionary Medicine.

Evolutionary Medicine

Evolution represents the unquestionable core concept of biological science (Grunspan et al. 2018). The introduction of evolution theory in natural science is inextricably associated with Charles Darwin, who published his fundamental work "On the Origin of Species by Means of Natural Selection," more than 160 years ago. Darwin is not only considered to be the founder of evolutionary theory, he also introduced terms such as evolution, selection, or survival of the fittest in natural science. Today, evolution is the central paradigm of biology and consequently, Theodosius Dobzhansky said that "*Nothing in biology makes sense except in the light of evolution*" (Dobzhansky 1973). In medical science however, the importance of an evolutionary perspective has been neglected for a long time. The term Evolutionary medicine was introduced in the early 1990s, mainly to explain the vulnerability to diseases today by means of evolutionary theory (Nesse & Stearns 2008). Nevertheless, evolutionary biology remains absent in most medical curricula up to now (Hidaka et al. 2015, Rühli et al. 2016), although Evolutionary Medicine is a rapidly growing field that applies the principles of evolutionary biology to health and disease. In particular, Evolutionary medicine tries to explain recent pathologies from an evolutionary viewpoint. Furthermore, the mismatch between our recent life style and our evolutionary heritage is focused on. Summarizing, the concept of Evolutionary medicine forced us to include an evolutionary perspective in medical science. Up to now, this evolutionary approach was only rarely applied on menopause associated complaints such as Climacteric symptomatology (Kirchengast & Rühli 2013, Froehle 2013).

Menopausal Transition - An Evolutionary Approach

From the viewpoint of evolutionary biology, the fact that human females lose their ability to reproduce quite early, is difficult to explain because it contradicts the concept of maximizing reproductive success and the biogenetic imperative (Dawkins 1976). Menopause is a biological phenomenon, and a universal one-time life event, which marks reproductive senescence among human females. A reduced probability of successful reproduction is found among several free-living social mammals such as toothed whales, elephants, lions or some primates (Nattrass 2018), an obligatory post-reproductive life stage of 30 years and more however, is exclusively found among recent human females (Wu et al. 2005). Current research indicates that menopause occurred first among *Homo erectus* who lived about 1.8 million years ago (Bogin 2020). At this stage of human evolution marked changes in life history patterns and life style occurred. Rapid encephalization resulted in larger brains, an important step on the way *to Homo sapiens.* Larger brains however, required larger skulls, even larger newborn skulls. Unfortunately, biomechanics of biped locomotion did not allow a widening of the bony pelvis. Therefore, the opposing evolutionary trends, biped locomotion and encephalization increased the risk of birth complications and resulted in the so-called obstetrical dilemma (Rosenberg & Trevanthan 1995). To make successful births possible, the evolutionary coping strategy was a decreased gestational period and the birth of immature helpless newborns. As a consequence, a long dependency of offspring and new life history patterns similar to those of recent *Homo sapiens* evolved (Bogin 2020). Furthermore, the phase of infancy decreased and weaning occurred earlier than among our closest relatives, the chimpanzees. In contrast to weaned chimpanzees, human children depend after weaning on older individuals for food and protection. This prolonged period of dependence makes extensive care, teaching and an especially high parental investment necessary (Hawkes et al. 1998). This support is mainly provided by the biological mothers however, mothers are often supported by so-called allomothers. Beside older siblings, first of all grandmothers or older female group members provide a substantial investment in young children (Hawkes et al. 1997, 1998. This is especially true of postmenopausal women with no young children of their own who help to feed and to take care of the offspring of their daughters and near relatives (Hawkes et al. 1998; Sear et al. 2000). This successful investment of postmenopausal women in related offspring, first of all grandchildren suggests a solution to the riddle of prolonged postmenopausal period in humans. The so-called grandmother hypothesis as an evolutionary explanation of female menopause was a consequence of such ideas (Hawkes et al. 1997; Hawkes 2003). Beside the grandmother hypothesis, several other evolutionary approaches such as the mother hypotheses, to explain the existence of menopause have been provided (Voland et al. 2005, Peccei 2001, Lahdenperä et al. 2004).

In contrast, to evolutionary basis of reproductive senescence, evolutionary interpretations of climacteric complaints are rare, because physiological or psychic symptoms associated with female reproductive senescence leave no traces on fossil bones. From the viewpoint of Evolutionary Medicine, climacteric complaints, but also cardiovascular disease, osteoporosis or postmenopausal breast cancer may be interpreted as results of a dramatic mismatch between our recent life style patterns and the environmental conditions we are adapted for. Currently, women are confronted with a late menopause associated with a rapid decline in estrogen levels. Female life history patterns of our ancestors however, were quite different and resembled those of contemporary hunter gatherer societies (Hawkes et al. 1997; Blurton Jones 2002). Women experienced low life time estrogen exposition, caused by a short reproductive span, late menarche, many pregnancies, long periods of lactation, and early menopause. On the other hand, daily physical activity was quite high. Therefore, we are neither adapted to the rapid decline of estrogen levels nor to low physically activity patterns typical of recent women in high-income countries. The consequence might be climacteric symptomatology, increased health risks and accelerated bone loss.

Physical Activity during Menopausal Transition

Currently, physical activity is increasingly seen as an alternative intervention for preventing or attenuating climacteric symptoms such as hot flushes but also psychological symptoms such as anxiety and depression (Pettree et al. 2015; Nelson et al. 2007, 2008; Sternfield & Dugan 2011). Several studies reported positive effects of physical activity during menopausal transition (Kim et al. 2014; Drabrowska-Galas et al. 2019; Khan et al. 2018; Pradanie et al. 2017). Physiologically, physical activity such as gymnastics, aerobics, but also walking may increase strength, flexibility and balance but also prevent osteoporosis and heart disease (Hu et al.2017). Regular resistance exercises, aerobic training and relaxation enhance satisfaction, avoid weight gain, prevent obesity, and decreases the risk of metabolic and cardiovascular diseases as well as cancer (Dabrowska-Galas et al. 2019, Daley et al. 2007). Furthermore, physical activity seems to have positive effects on cartilage and bones, and reduces in this way the risk of osteoporosis. Dabrowska-Galas et al. (2019) reported severe somato-vegetative symptoms among menopausal women with low physical activity levels, while women with high and moderate physical activity levels show less severe climacteric symptoms in comparison to inactive ones. Although the results of many studies plead for positive effects of physical activity on climacteric complaints and general well-being, and exercise has been recommended as a strategy to reduce climacteric symptoms, in particular hot flushes or night sweats, several studies yielded no association between physical activity and the degree of severity of the climacteric syndrome (Daley et al. 2015). While physical activity improves quality of life scores, no effects of physical activity on climacteric symptoms such as hot flushes were reported (Daley et al. 2007, 2015; Elavsky &McAuley 2007). According to the Cochrane review of exercise for the management of vasomotor menopausal symptoms, increased physical activity seems not to be an effective treatment for hot flushes and other vasomotor climacteric complaints (Daley et al. 2015).

An unquestionable positive effect of physical activity is the reduced risk of obesity and associated cardiovascular and metabolic symptoms (Dabrowska et al.2015). A moderate or high physical activity reduces the amount of adipose tissue or prevent an increase of adipose tissue. A lower amount of adipose tissue is associated with lower estrogen levels during menopausal transition and postmenopause because the aromatization of androgens to estrogens takes place in adipose tissue cells (Cohen 2001) Consequently, physical activity during menopausal transition and during postmenopause is associated with lower levels of estrogens. Lower levels of circulating estrogens reduce the risk of breast and endometrium cancer during this phase of life. A sedentary life style characterized by low physical activity in contrast, is associated with higher estrogen levels, a higher amount of adipose tissue, an increased risk of obesity and as a consequence a n increased risk of cancer and metabolic as well as cardiovascular diseases (Dabrowska et al. 2015).

Another menopause associated health problem is bone loss, which accelerates after menopause. A reduction of bone mass of 0.6%, 1.1%, and 2.1% per year was reported for the age groups 60 to 69 years, 70 to79 years, and 80 age and beyond (Gomez-Cabello et al. 2012). Therefore, the effects of physical activity patterns on bone health were discussed too. Although exercise is widely recommended as an appropriate strategy to reduce the risk of osteoporosis, its effects on bone are controversial. Current guidelines for strategies to prevent and treat osteoporosis, recommend physical exercise as an effective strategy to maintain bone mass and bone density, but also to reduce bone loss throughout menopausal transition, postmenopause and during old age (Santos et al. 2017), however, a positive skeletal response is not equally found for all kinds and frequencies of exercise training. According to Wolff´s law and Frost´s mechanostat model physical activity may have a positive impact on bone formation, bone structure and consequently on bone health. On the other hand, low or non-impact aerobic activities, such as swimming or walking have only small positive effects bone loss after menopause (Ma et al. 2013). This may be due to the insufficient levels of loads on bones associated with these leisure time exercise activities. During young age exercise has a clear positive effect on bone mass and bone size (Ma et al. 2013), among elderly people physical activity does not increase bone mass, but may increase bone density and resistance of cortical bone at loaded skeletal areas (Kohrt et al. 2004). In addition to the positive effects of physical activity on bone health, physical activity avoids the reduction of skeletal muscle mass with increasing age. Inactivity and a sedentary life style have tremendous effects on skeletal muscle mass. In 1989, Rosenberg introduced the term sarcopenia to describe the progressive loss of muscle mass and muscle strength with increasing age (Rosenberg 1989). A lack of training and physical inactivity contributes to the development of sarcopenia and the so-called frailty syndrome, while in contrast, physical activity not only avoid muscle loss, but also increase muscle mass and muscle strength, even among elderly people (Messier et al. 2011). Increased muscle strength does not only prevent frailty associated falls and in this way fatal fractures, it also enhances health related quality of life (Musalek & Kichengast 2017). Therefore, physical activity during middle ages and beyond seems to reduce various health risks and to have positive effects on well-being.

PHYSICAL ACTIVITY DURING MENOPAUSAL TRANSITION – AN EVOLUTIONARY APPROACH

Although the effects of physical activity patterns on climacteric complaints are discussed controversial, there is no doubt that physical activity helps to prevent several menopause-associated health risks, such as obesity, metabolic and cardiovascular disorders but also estrogen associated cancers and bone loss and sarcopenia in later life. From the viewpoint of Evolutionary Medicine, these positive effects of physical activity are expected because *Homo sapiens* is clearly adapted to a highly active life style. The menopause associated health risks mentioned above are mainly the result of a mismatch between our contemporary life style and our evolutionary heritage. According to Williams and Nesse (1991) our bodies are designed for Stone Age conditions, but are not well adapted to our current environment. We all are members of the genus *Homo*, which first appeared nearly 2.5 million years ago (Henke & Hardt 2011). The daily life of our ancestors was characterized by an extraordinary high degree of physical activity. This was mainly due to the fact, that physical activity was essential for surviving in the harsh habitat of the African savanna. Predators, hunger and thirst forced our ancestors to follow a physically active lifestyle. Hunting and gathering, looking for shelter and water resources required walking - and sometimes running - long distances. These daily activity patterns have been typical of 99% of our evolutionary history (Eaton et al. 1988).

Until about 10 000 years ago, *Homo sapiens* depended on subsistence patterns characterized by high mobility and a generally high degree of physical activity. In order to collect vegetabile foods, but also to look for a new base camp or water whole, people had to move around for hours every day. In addition, women had to carry their children for long distances until they were about 4 years old (Eaton et al. 1988). High physical activity was an essential factor to survive, consequently, the physically active life style of our ancestors was not motivated by the desire of leisure time activities, physical activity was the key factor to avoid hunger, thirst and danger (Walker et al. 2003). Similar patterns of daily physical activities were found up to now among the few remaining contemporary hunter gatherer populations such as the Hadza in Tanzania, the !Kung of Namibia and Botswana, Ache of Paraguay or Efe of central Africa (Kirchengast 2014).

Regular physical activity has clearly positive effects on bone mass and bone size during childhood, adolescence and early adulthood. Bone mass is increasing during the first three decades of life resulting in the peak bone mass which is achieved between the ages 25 and 30 years. Peak bone mass, however has long-term effects on bone health. Unfortunately, our recent life style is characterized by an extraordinary low rate of physical activity from early childhood onwards. Today, it is not necessary to run, to climb up trees or even to walk in order to hunt or gather.

Up to the 20th century, daily life was still characterized by hard work and high levels of physical activity. During the last 140 years a dramatic change occurred and the vast majority of recent humans are confronted with an environment which is completely different from that in which our species evolved. In westernized countries, we live in urban environments characterized by a sophisticated technology, sedentary jobs, labor-saving household technologies and consequently no need for regular physical activity in daily life. Only few individuals are motivated to be physically active during leisure time, while spending leisure time by watching TV or surfing in the internet is a preferred leisure time activity.

This lifestyle is completely new in our evolution. How are these life style changes related to our topic menopause and physical activity?

A clear positive association between physical activity and bone mass and bone density could be stated. Our ancestors had to follow a physically highly active life style from early childhood onwards. Physical activity during the subadult phase and early adulthood has a positive long-term effect on bone mass and bone density. Furthermore, high levels of physical activity persist up to old age. An osteological indicator of physical activity patterns of our paleolithic ancestors is their high skeletal robustness (Ryan & Shaw 2015). In addition, there is no evidence for osteoporosis among upper paleolithic skeletal remains. We can assume, that even among postmenopausal females a high level of daily physical activity might have prevent them from accelerated bone loss and osteoporosis. Kirsten Hawkes pointed out the extraordinary high physical activity among postmenopausal Hadza women (Hawkes et al. 1997). Reduced bone density, osteoporosis or increased fracture rates are not observed among this contemporary hunter gatherer society.

Furthermore, there is no doubt, that physical activity reduces the risk of cardiovascular and metabolic diseases. The analyses of health and disease patterns among the few remaining contemporary hunter gatherer population or traditional societies reveal a very low prevalence of obesity, cardiovascular or metabolic diseases. High physical activity and traditional nutritional habits characterized by a high amount of lean meat, fiber, wild vegetables, tubers, berries, fruits, nuts and roots and a low amount of fat and carbohydrates are typical life style patterns. The positive effects of high physical activity and these dietary habits on weight status, metabolic and cardiovascular symptoms are unquestionable. But why does physical activity not have such a definitive positive effect on climacteric symptomatology?

The main problem seems to be, that physical activity as a treatment of climacteric complaints often starts too late, i.e., during menopausal transition or postmenopause, when suffering from climacteric complaints makes life stressful and uncomfortable. Of course, better late than never, but from an evolutionary viewpoint we are adapted to a highly physically active lifestyle from childhood onwards. The recent strategy to start with physical activity to reduce climacteric complaints or to prevent osteoporosis during late adulthood, seems to be quite late. Without any doubt, physically activity even starting late has many positive effects on body weight, well-being and quality of life, it also may reduce climacteric complaints, a better strategy however would be to start as early as possible with regular physical activity and to incorporate physical activity in daily life and leisure time from childhood onwards (Santos et al. 2017; Langsetmo et al. 2012). This strategy may help to increase bone density and bone mass during young age and reduce age dependent bone loss during middle and old age. Furthermore, the risk of metabolic and cardiovascular diseases as well as cancer may be reduced. In addition, a positive effect on climacteric symptomatology is possible. From an evolutionary perspective, this strategy is a completely new challenge for *Homo sapiens*, because the first time in our evolution and history we have to be physical active not for looking for shelter or food, but for staying healthy.

References

Austad, S. N. 1997. Postreproductive survival. In Wachter, K. W., and Finch, C. E. (eds.) *Between Zeus and the Salmon: the Biodemography of Longevity*, National Academy Press, Washington, D.C., pp. 161–174.

Beyene, Y. 1986. Cultural significance and physiological manifestations of menopause: A biocultural analysis. *Culture Medicine Psychiatry* 10: 47-71.

Blurton Jones, N. G., Hawkes, K., O´Connell, J. F. 2002. Antiquity of postreproductive life. Are there modern impacts on hunter gatherer postreproductive life spans? *American Journal of Human Biology* 14:184-202.

Bogin, B. 2020. *Patterns of human growth*, Cambridge University Press, Cambridge.

Bojar, I., Lyubinets, O., Novotny, J., Stanchak, Y., Tiszczenko, E., Owoc, A., Raczkiewicz, D. 2016. Intensification of menopausal symptoms among female inhabitants of East European countries. *Annals Agriculture Environmental Medicine* 23:517-24.

Burger, H. G., Hale, G. E., Robertson, D. M., Dennerstein, L. 2007. A review of hormonal changes during the menopausal transition: focus on findings from the Melbourne Women's Midlife Health project. *Human Reproduction Update* 13: 559-565.

Cohen, P.G. 2001. Aromatase, adiposity, aging and disease. The hypogonadal-metabolic-atherogenic-disease and aging connection. *Medical Hypotheses* 56:702-8.

Dąbrowska, J., Dąbrowska-Galas, M., Naworska, B., Wodarska, M., & Plinta, R. 2015. The role of physical activity in preventing obesity in midlife women. *Menopause review*, 14: 13–19. https://doi.org/10.5114/pm.2015.49252.

Dabrowska-Galas, M., Dabrowska, J., Ptaszkowski, K., Plinta, R. 2019. High physical activity level may reduce menopausal symptoms. *Medicina* 55: doi.10.3390/medicina55080466.

Daley, A. J., MacArthur, C., Stokes-Lampard, H., McManus, R., Wilson, S., Mutri, N. 2007. Exercise participation, body mass index and health related quality of life in women of menopausal age. *British Journal General Practice* 57: 130-135.

Daley, A. J., Thomas, A., Roalfe, A. K., Stokes-Lampard, H., Coleman, S., Rees, M., Hunter, M. S., MacArthur, C. 2015. The effectiveness of exercise as treatment for vasomotor menopausal symptoms: randomized controlled trial. *BJOG* 12: 565-575.

Davis, S., Lambrinoudaki, I., Lumsden, M., Mishra, G. D., Pal, L., Rees, M., Santoro, N., Simoncini, T. 2015. Menopause. *Nature Reviews Disease Primers* 1, 15004 https://doi.org/10.1038/nrdp.2015.4.

Dobzhansky, T. 1973. Nothing in Biology makes sense except in the light of evolution. *The American Teacher* 35: 125-129.

Dawkins, R. (1976): *The selfish gene* Oxford: Oxford University Press.

Eaton, S. B., Konner, M., Shostak, M. 1988. Stone agers in the fast lane; chronic degenerative diseases in evolutionary perspective. *American Journal of Medicine* 84: 739-749.

Eaton, S. B., Pike, M. C., Short, R. V., Lee, N. C., Trussell, J., Hatcher, R. A., Wood, J. W., Worthman, C. M., Nicolas, G. B. I., Konner, M. J., Bailey, R., Hurtado, A. M. 1994. Women's reproductive cancers in evolutionary context. *Quarterly Review Biology* 69: 353-3657.

Elavsky, S., McAuley, E. 2007. Physical activity and mental health outcomes during menopause: a randomized controlled trial. *Annals Behavioral Medicine* 33: 132-142.

Fait, T. 2019. Menopause hormone therapy: latest developments and clinical practice. *Drugs in context* 8: 212551. https://doi.org/10.7573/dic.212551.

Froehle, A. W. 2013. Postmenopausal Health and Disease from the Perspective of Evolutionary Medicine. *Anthropology & Ageing* 34: 61-86.

Gold, E. B. 2011. The timing of the age at which natural menopause occurs. *Obstetrics Gynecology Clinics North America* 38: 425-440.

Gómez-Cabello, A., Ara, I., González-Agüero, A., Casajús, J. A., Vicente-Rodríguez, G. 2012. Effects of training on bone mass in older adults: a systematic review. *Sports Medicine* 42:301–325.

Grunspan, D. Z., Nesse, R. M., Barnes, M. E., Brownell, S. E. 2018. Core principles of evolutionary medicine: A Delphi study, *Evolution, Medicine, and Public Health* 1: 13–23, https://doi.org/10.1093/emph/eox025.

Hawkes, K., O´Connell, J. F., Blurton, Jones N. G. 1997. Hadza women ´s time allocation, offspring provisioning and the evolution of long postmenopausal lifespans. *Current Anthropology* 38: 551-577.

Hawkes, K., O´Connell, J. F., Blurton Jones, N. G., Alvarez, H., Charnov, A. L. 1998. Grandmothering, menopause and the evolution of human life histories. *Proceeding of the National Academy of Science* 95: 1336-1339.

Hawkes, K. 2003. Grandmothering of human longevity. *American Journal of Human Biology*15: 380-400.

Henke, W.; Hardt, T. The genus *Homo*: origin, speciation and dispersal, in: S.Condemi, G.-C.Weniger (Eds.), Continuity and Discontinuity in the peopling of Europe: One hundred fifty years of Neanderthal study, *Vertebrate Paleobiology and Paleoanthropology*. Springer Press, New York, 2011, pp. 17-43.

Hidaka, B. H., Asghar, A., Aktipis, C. A., 2015. The status of evolutionary medicine education in North American medical schools *BMC Medical Education* 5: 38.

Hu, L., Zhu, L., Lyu, J., Zho, W., Xu, Y., Yang, L. 2017. Benefits of walking on menopausal symptoms and mental health outcomes among Chinese postmenopausal women. *International Journal Gerontology* 11: 166-170.

Khan, B. E. Z., Rahman, A. M., Begum, N., Halim, K. S., Muna, A. T., Mostary, K. F., Islam, M. S. 2018. Physical activity and menopausal symptoms. *Bangladesh Medical Journal* 47: 11-17.

Kim, M. J., Cho, J., Ahn, Y., Yim, G., Park, H. Y. 2014. Association between physical activity and menopausal symptoms in perimenopausal women. *Women's Health* 14: 122-129.

Kirchengast, S. Physical inactivity from the viewpoint of evolutionary medicine. *Sports* 2: 34-50.

Kirchengast, S., Huber, J. 2012. Sex specific associations between soft tissue body composition and bone mineral density among older adults. *Annals of Human Biology* 39: 206.

Kirchengast, S., Rühli, F. Evolutionary medicine and its implications for endocrinological issues (e.g., menopause). *Comparative Endocrinology* 2186:145-149.

Kirchengast, S., Gruber, D., Sator, M., Hartmann, B., Knogler, W., Huber, J. 1997. Menopause associated differences in female fat patterning estimated by dual-energy-x-ray absorptiometry. *Annals of Human Biology* 24: 45-54.

Kohrt, W. M., Bloomfield, S. A., Little, K. D., Nelson, M. E., Yingling, V. R. 2004. Physical activity and bone health. *Medicine & Science in Sports & Exercise.* 36:1985–1996.

Lahdenperä, M., Lummaa, V., Helle, S., Tremblay, M., Russell, A. F. 2004. Fitness benefits of prolonged post-reproductive lifespan in women. *Nature* 428: 178-181.

Langsetmo, L., Hichcock, C.L., Kingwell, E.J., Davison, K.S., Berger, C., Forsmo, S., Zhou, W., Kreiger, N., Prior, J.C. 2012. Physical activity, body mass index and bone mineral density – associations in a prospective population-based cohort of women and men: The Canadian Multicentre osteoporosis study (CaMos) *Bone* 50: 401-408

Leidy-Sievert, L. 2006. *Menopause. A biocultural perspective*, Rutgers University Press, London.

Lukács, A., Horváth, E., Máté, Z., Szabo, A.; Virag, K., Papp, M., Sandor, J., Adany, R.; Pauli, E. 2019. Abdominal obesity increases metabolic risk factors in non-obese adults: a Hungarian cross-sectional study. *BMC Public Health* 19, 1533 https://doi.org/10.1186/s12889-019-7839-1.

Lumsden, M. A. 2016. The NICE Guideline – Menopause: diagnosis and management, *Climacteric*, 19: 426-429, DOI: 10.1080/13697137.2016.1222483.

Ma, D., Wu, L., He, Z. 2013. Effects of walking on the preservation of bone mineral density in perimenopausal and postmenopausal women: a systematic review and meta-analysis. *Menopause* 20:1216–1226.

McCrea, F. B. 1983. The politics of menopause: The discovery of a deficiency disease. *Social Problems* 31: 111-123.

Melby, M. K.; Lock, M.; Kaufert, P. 2005. Culture and symptom reporting at menopause, *Human Reproduction Update*, 11: 495–512.

Messier, V., Rahbasa-Lhoret, R., Barbat-Artigas, S., Elisha, B., Kargelis, A. D., Aubertin-Leheurdre, M. 2011. Menopause and sarcopenia: A potential role for sex hormones. *Maturitas* 68: 331-336.

Monteleone, P., Mascagni, G., Giannini, A., Genazzani A. R., Simoncini, T. 2018. Symptoms of menopause — global prevalence, physiology and implications. *National Review Endocrinology* 14: 199–215 https://doi.org/10.1038/nrendo.2017.180.

Musalek, C., Kirchengast, S. 2017. Grip Strength as an Indicator of Health-Related Quality of Life in Old Age-A Pilot Study. *International Journal of Environmental Research and Public Health* 14:1447.

Narod, S. A. 2011. Hormone replacement therapy and the risk of breast cancer. *National Review Clinical Oncology* 8:669-76.

Nattrass, S., Croft, D. P., Ellis, S., Cant, M. A., Weiss, M. N., Wright, B. M., Stredulinsky, E., Doniol-Valcroze, T., Ford, J. K. B., Balcomb, K. C., Franks, D. W. 2019. Postreproductive killer whale grandmothers improve the survival of their grandoffspring. *Proceedings of the National Academy of Sciences* 116: 26669-26673; DOI: 10.1073/pnas.1903844116.

Nelson, D. B., Sammel, M. D., Freeman, E. W., Lin, H., Gracia, C. R., Schmitz, K. H. 2008. Effect of physical activity on menopausal symptoms among urban women. *Medical Science Sports Exercise* 40: 50-58.

Nelson, M. E., Rejeski, W. J., Blair, S. N. 2007. Physical activity and public health in older adults: recommendation from the American College of Sports Medicine and the American Heart Association. *Circulation* 116:1094–1105.

Nesse, R. M., Stearns, S. C. 2008. The great opportunity: Evolutionary applications to medicine and public health. *Evolutionary Applications* 1: 28-48.

Palacios, S., Henderson, V. W., Siseles, N., Tan, D., Viööaseca, P. 2010. Age of menopause and impact of climacteric symptoms by geographical region. *Climacteric* 13: 419-428.

Peccei, J. S. 2001. Menopause: Adaptation or Epiphenomenon? *Evolutionary Anthropology* 12: 43-57.

Pettree Gabriel K. P., Mason J. M., Sternfeld B. 2015. Recent evidence exploring the associations between physical activity and menopausal symptoms in midlife women: perceived risks and possible health benefits. *Women's Midlife Health* 1: doi.org/10.1186/s40695-015-0004-91.

Pradanie, R., Maràh, Has, E. M., Malichah, T. 2017. Correlation of physical activity and menopause symptoms. *Advances Health Research* 3: 152-156.

Pu, D., Tan, R., Yu, Q., Wu, J. 2017. Metabolic syndrome in menopause and associated factors: a meta-analysis, *Climacteric* 20: 583-591, DOI: 10.1080/13697137.2017.1386649.

Rosenberg, I. H. 1989. Epidemiologic and methodologic problems in determining nutritional-status of older persons. *American Journal of Clinical Nutrition*. 50:1231–1233.

Rosenberg K., Trevathan W. 1995. Bipedalism and human birth: The obstetrical dilemma revisited. *Evolutionary Anthropology* 4: 161-168.

Rühli, F., Haeusler, M., Saniotis, A., Henneberg, M. 2016. Novel Modules to Teach Evolutionary Medicine: an Australian and a Swiss

Experience. *Medical Science Education* 26: 375–381 https://doi.org/10.1007/s40670-016-0245-8.

Ryan, T.M., Shaw, C.N. 2015. Gracility of the modern Homo sapiens skeleton is the result of decreased biomechanical loading *Proceeding of the National Academy of Science* 112: 372-377.

Sear, R., Mace, R., McGregor, I. A. 2000. Maternal grandmothers improve nutritional status and survival of children in rural Gambia. *Proceedings Royal Society London Series* B 267: 1641-1647.

Santos, L., Elliott-Sale, K. J., Sale, C. 2017. Exercise and bone health across the lifespan. *Biogerontology* 18: 931-946.

Sheikholeslami S, Ghanbarian A, Azizi F. 2018. The Impact of Physical Activity on Non-communicable Diseases: Findings from 20 Years of the Tehran Lipid and Glucose Study. *International Journal of Endocrinology and Metabolism* 16: e84740. doi: 10.5812/ijem.84740.

Stachowiak, G., Pertyński, T., & Pertyńska-Marczewska, M. (2015). Metabolic disorders in menopause. *Przeglad menopauzalny = Menopause review*, 14: 59–64. https://doi.org/10.5114/pm.2015.50000.

Sternfeld, B., Dugan, S. 2011. Physical activity and health during menopausal transition. *Obstetrics Gynecology Clinical North America* 38: 537-566.

Sussman, M., Trocio, J., Best, C. Mirkin, D. S., Bushmakin, A. G., Yood, R., Friedman, M., Menzin, J., Louie, M. 2015. Prevalence of menopausal symptoms among mid-life women: findings from electronic medical records. *BMC Women's Health* 15, 58. https://doi.org/10.1186/s12905-015-0217-y.

Tella, S. H., & Gallagher, J. C. 2014. Prevention and treatment of postmenopausal osteoporosis. *The Journal of steroid biochemistry and molecular biology*, *142*, 155–170. https://doi.org/10.1016/j.jsbmb.2013.09.008.

Van de Wiel, L. 2014. The time of the change: Menopause's medicalization and the gender politics of aging. *International Journal Feminist Approach Bioethics* 7: 74-98.

Voland E., Chasiotis A., Schiefenhövel W. Grandmotherhood. 2005. *The evolutionary significance of the second half of female life*. Rutgers University Press. New York.

Walker, A. R. P., Walker, B. F., Adam, F. 2003. Nutrition, diet, physical activity, smoking and longevity: from primitive hunter gatherer to present passive consumer – how far can we go? *Nutrition* 19: 169-173.

Williams, G. C., Nesse, R. M. 1991. The dawn of Darwinian medicine. *Quarterly Reviews Biology* 66: 1-22.

Woods, N. F., Mitchell, E. S. 2005. Symptoms during the perimenopause: prevalence, severity, trajectory, and significance in women's lives. *American Journal of Medicine*118 (Suppl 12B):14–24.

Wu, J. M., Zelinski, M. B., Ingram, D. K., Ottinger, M. A. 2005. Ovarian Ageing and menopause: current theories, hypotheses and research models. *Experimental Biology Medicine* 230: 818-828.

INDEX

D

E

F

G

H

I

K

L

M

N

O

P

T

U

V

W

Y